LUMBAR SPINE DISORDERS

Current Concepts

LUMBAR
SPINE
DISORDERS
Current Concepts

Editors

R. M. Aspden
R. W. Porter

Department of Orthopaedic Surgery
University of Aberdeen

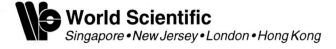 **World Scientific**
Singapore • New Jersey • London • Hong Kong

Published by

World Scientific Publishing Co. Pte. Ltd.

P O Box 128, Farrer Road, Singapore 9128

USA office: Suite 1B, 1060 Main Street, River Edge, NJ 07661

UK office: 57 Shelton Street, Covent Garden, London WC2H 9HE

LUMBAR SPINE DISORDERS: CURRENT CONCEPTS

ISBN: 981-02-2175-4

Printed in Singapore.

Great are the works of the Lord,
Studied by all who have pleasure in them.
                              Psalm 111

CONTENTS

Page

Acknowledgements   xi

Preface   xiii

Contributors   xv

Chapter 1
The curved, flexible spine and the functions of ligaments and muscles   1
R.M. Aspden

Chapter 2
Forces acting on the lumbar spine   15
P. Dolan and M.A. Adams

Chapter 3
What is lumbar instability?   26
D.W.L. Hukins

Chapter 4
Towards a logical basis for the design of spinal implants   38
J. Dove

Chapter 5
**Biomechanics of the intervertebral disc - disc pressure
measurements and significance**   42
D.S. McNally

Chapter 6
**The extracellular matrix of the intervertebral disc:
proteoglycan biochemistry**   51
B. Johnstone and M.T. Bayliss

Chapter 7
**The effect of mechanical stress on cellular activity
in the intervertebral disc**   63
J.P.G. Urban and K. Puustjarvi

Chapter 8
**The microanatomy of intervertebral tissues
in the normal and scoliotic spine**   73
S. Roberts

Chapter 9
Neuropeptides in the lumbar spine   85
I.K. Ashton and S.M. Eisenstein

Chapter 10
Growth and development of the lumbar vertebral canal   97
R.W. Porter

Chapter 11
Pathological changes contributing to back pain and sciatica   105
J.A.N. Shepperd

Chapter 12
**Measurement of vertebral blood flow and its
significance in disc disease**   115
A.M.C. Thomas, G.F. Keenan and M. Brown

Chapter 13
The pathophysiology of neurogenic claudication   120
R.W. Porter

Chapter 14
**The role of vascular damage in the development
of nerve root problems**   132
M.I.V. Jayson and A.J. Freemont

Chapter 15
The assessment of the patient with low back pain   145
C.D. Greenough

Chapter 16
**Fear-avoidance: the natural history of back pain
and its management**   155
J.D.G. Troup and P.D. Slade

Chapter 17
Chemonucleolysis   164
M. Sullivan

Chapter 18
Experience with chemonucleolysis   167
D. Wardlaw

Chapter 19
Lumbo-sacral and spondylo-pelvic arthrodesis   185
A.D.H. Gardner

Chapter 20
Radical resection of vertebral body tumours:
a surgical technique used in ten cases   209
M.W. Fidler

Chapter 21
Costs and effectiveness:
approaches to the management of back pain   225
J.A.K. Moffett and G. Richardson

Index   237

Acknowledgements

We wish to acknowledge the support of Action Research who enabled the University of Aberdeen to establish the Sir Harry Platt Chair of Orthopaedic Surgery and the academic Department of Orthopaedic Surgery. We are also grateful to the Arthritis and Rheumatism Council, the Wellcome Trust, the Colt Foundation, the Sir Jules Thorn Charitable Trust and the National Back Pain Association who have funded our spine research in the Department. Our thanks must go too to Molly Russell who laboured hard over this book to ensure a uniformity of style and accuracy. The responsibility for any errors of presentation that remain must lie with ourselves.

Preface

This anniversary book on 'Back pain' celebrates an important occasion, the quincentenary of Aberdeen University. In 1495 Bishop Elphinstone won the support of King James IV to provide a centre of learning in the North. Besides a University which would produce priests, schoolmasters and lawyers, James, who dabbled in medicine, may well have been Elphinstone's encourager to provide for the teaching of medicine and surgery. Playing to the remoteness of northern Scotland, he suggested that the inhabitants were "rude, ignorant of letters, almost barbarians" and were worthy of Britain's first medical school.

Now the capital oil-city of Europe, Aberdeen boasts of a prosperous economy, and a thriving University. And this year also celebrates another anniversary - the fifth year of the founding of the University Department of Orthopaedics. Our strong interest in disorders of the lumbar spine has prompted us to compile an anniversary book on "Back Pain Disorders", inviting contributions from friends around the UK who have done valuable research in this area. They come from many disciplines, basic scientists, physicians and surgeons, to share the results of their research on the most common of medical disorders. The outcome is deliberately personal and no attempt has been made to reconcile the differing views presented. This is meant to be provocative and reflects both the extent of our ignorance and the amount of active work that is still in progress. In order to be topical this book has been produced to a very tight schedule. Inevitably, therefore, we have overlooked one or two names that ought to be included and some, due to pressure of other commitments, have been unable to prepare something in the time we gave them. To these people we apologise, but maybe this gives us scope for a second edition!

One might ask why has back pain disability increased three fold in the past twenty years, when it has been the subject of so much excellent research? We know so much more about the structure of the spine, its physiology, and pathological change. We understand how discs become degenerate, and the complex changes that take place with neurological compromise. We have improved clinical skills, and better imaging. Our therapy is more refined. Surgical skills have improved, helped by impressive implant technology. Why then is back pain disability getting worse?

It is hardly possible that the environment is to blame. With such interest in ergonomics, the creation of a safe environment, and regulations on safe work handling, backs can not be suffering from greater mechanical stresses. Nor is it likely that in the workplace we now have a cohort of individuals with particularly weak backs. For the cause of increased disability we must focus rather on society and the socio-economic climate. Although the science is undoubtedly improving, chronic disability will flourish in a climate of low self-esteem, and broken relationships. These are beyond our immediate remit, but might be areas of productive research for a millennial volume. However enjoy the science, and muse on the answers to a major health problem. Perhaps we are still "rude, ignorant of letters, and almost barbarians".

CONTRIBUTORS

M.A. Adams, PhD
Research Fellow
Comparative Orthopaedic Research Unit
Department of Anatomy
University of Bristol
Southwell Street
Bristol
BS2 8EJ.

I.K. Ashton
The Robert Jones and Agnes Hunt
Orthopaedic and District Hospital NHS
Trust
Oswestry
Shropshire
SY10 7AG

R.M. Aspden, PhD
Medical Research Council Senior Fellow
University of Aberdeen
Department of Orthopaedic Surgery
Polwarth Building
Foresterhill
Aberdeen
AB9 2ZD

M.T. Bayliss, PhD
Senior Researcher
Division of Biochemistry
The Kennedy Institute of Rheumatology
Hammersmith
London W6 7DW

M. Brown, PhD
Research Fellow
Department of Physiology
University of Birmingham
The Medical School
Birmingham
B15 2TJ

P. Dolan, PhD
Research Fellow
Comparative Orthopaedic Research Unit
Department of Anatomy
University of Bristol
Southwell Street
Bristol
BS2 8EJ.

J. Dove, FRCS
Consultant Orthopaedic Surgeon
Stoke-on-Trent Spinal Service
31 Quarry Avenue
Hartshill
Stoke-on-Trent
ST4 7EW

S.M. Eisenstein, PhD, FRCS(Ed)
Consultant Orthopaedic Surgeon
The Robert Jones and Agnes Hunt
Orthopaedic and District Hospital NHS
Trust
Oswestry
Shropshire
SY10 7AG

M.W. Fidler, MS, FRCS
Consultant Orthopaedic Surgeon
Onze Lieve Vrouwe Gasthuis
Postbus 95500
1090 HM Amsterdam
The Netherlands

A.J. Freemont, MD, MRCPath, FRCP(Ed)
Professor of Osteoarticular Pathology
Department of Rheumatology
University of Manchester
Stopford Building
Oxford Road
Manchester M13 9PT

A.D.H. Gardner, FRCS
Senior Consultant Orthopaedic Surgeon
Essex Spine Centre,
BUPA Hartswood Hospital,
Brentwood, Essex, UK

C. Greenough, MD, FRCS
Consultant Orthopaedic Surgeon
Department of Orthopaedic Surgery
Middlesborough General Hospital
Ayrsome Green Lane
Middlesborough
Cleveland
TS5 5AZ

D.W.L. Hukins, DSc, PhD
MacRobert Professor of Physics
University of Aberdeen
Department of Bio-Medical Physics and
Bioengineering
Foresterhill
Aberdeen
AB9 2ZD

M.I.V. Jayson, MD, FRCP
Professor of Rheumatology
Rheumatic Diseases Centre
Clinical Sciences Building
Hope Hospital
Eccles Old Road
Salford M6 8HD

B. Johnstone, PhD
Department of Orthopaedics
Case Western Reserve University
Cleveland
Ohio
USA

G.F. Keenan, FRCS
Career Orthopaedic Registrar
Department of Orthopaedic Surgery
Aberdeeen Royal Hopitals (NHS) Trust
Foresterhill
Aberdeen AB9 2ZD

D.S. McNally, PhD
Lecturer
Department of Anatomy
University of Bristol
School of Veterinary Science
Southwell Street
Bristol
BS2 8EJ

J.A.K. Moffett, PhD, MCSP
Research Fellow
Centre for Health Economics
University of York
Heslington
York
YO1 5DD

R.W. Porter, MD, FRCS, FRCSE
Sir Harry Platt Professor of Orthopaedic
Surgery
University of Aberdeen
Department of Orthopaedic Surgery
Polwarth Building
Foresterhill
Aberdeen
AB9 2ZD

K. Puustjarvi, PhD, MD
Research Fellow
University of Oxford
University Laboratory of Physiology
Parks Road
Oxford
OX1 3PT

G. Richardson
Research Fellow
Centre for Health Economics
University of York
Heslington
York
YO1 5DD

S. Roberts, PhD
Research Fellow
Centre for Spinal studies -Oswestry
Robert Jones and Agnes Hunt
Orthopaedic and District Hospital NHS
Trust
Oswestry
Shropshire
SY10 7AG

J.A.N. Shepperd, FRCS
Consultant Orthopaedic Surgeon
The Directorate of Orthopaedic Surgery
and Accident and Emergency Medicine
Conquest Hospital
The Ridge
St. Leonards-on-Sea
East Sussex
TN37 7RD

P.D. Slade, PhD
Professor
Department of Clinical Psychology
University of Liverpool
P.O. Box 147
Liverpool
L69 3BX

M.F. Sullivan, FRCS
Consultanat Orthopaedic Surgeon
95 Harley Street
London W1N 1DF

A.M.C. Thomas, FRCS
Consultant Orthopaedic Surgeon
Royal Orthopaedic Hospital Birmingham
The Medical School
Birminham
B15 2TJ

**J.D.G. Troup, PhD, DSc(Med),
MRCS, LRCP, M(FOM)RCP, FergS**
Honorary Senior Research Fellow
Department of Orthopaedic Surgery
University of Aberdeen
Polwarth Building
Foresterhill
Aberdeen
Ab9 2ZD

J.P.G. Urban, PhD
Arthritis and Rheumatism Council Senior
Fellow
University of Oxford
University Laboratory of Physiology
Parks Road
Oxford
OX1 3PT

D. Wardlaw, ChM, FRCSE
Consultant Orthopaedic Surgeon
Department of Orthopaedic Surgery
Aberdeeen Royal Hopitals (NHS) Trust
Foresterhill
Aberdeen
AB9 2ZD

CHAPTER 1

THE CURVED, FLEXIBLE SPINE AND THE FUNCTIONS
OF LIGAMENTS AND MUSCLES

R.M. Aspden

1. Introduction

The spine forms the most complicated supportive structure in the human body. Its strength and flexibility combine to enable considerable loads to be carried in a wide variety of postures. How it does this is still a matter of considerable research activity and debate. Some of this debate can be seen in the next chapter in which the more traditional approach is adopted to understand the biomechanical behaviour of the spine. In this chapter I shall show how the curved, flexible nature of the spine enables it to function as an arch-like structure and how this provides an explanation for the complexity of the muscles and ligaments which make up the spine. First, I shall explain why modelling of the spine is important and how different models lead to very different conclusions regarding its behaviour. I shall show that the arch model provides a consistent description of the properties of the spine and its mechanical function by making full use of the natural curvature and flexibility. Implicit in the concept of the arch is the corollary that the muscles and ligaments form an intrinsic part of the spine; they are not separate agents acting externally to stabilise an otherwise unstable structure. Recent descriptions of the ligaments and the muscular anatomy will then be surveyed to demonstrate how the subtleties and complexities of organisation that have been described are required to enable proper function of the structure as a whole.

2. Modelling the spine

What is the purpose of modelling a structure such as the spine? What relationship does the model have with reality? A model of any complicated system should simplify the system so that its behaviour can be more clearly understood but without losing any of the essential features. A model that is too simple may enable a first description of the behaviour to be made but one that is found not to predict or explain all the phenomena that are subsequently observed. Conversely, too detailed a model may not be a simplification at all but merely result in exchanging one set of complexities for another. The traditional model of the spine, that based on a system of levers, is increasingly being found to fall into the first category. It provides an easily understandable concept and a simple method of analysis but its predictions are less and less believable. The model has its origins in attempts to estimate the forces developed in the spine when lifting[1] and has developed significantly since those early, very simple, approximations. The basic assumption behind the model is that bending moments generated by lifting a weight in front of the body are balanced directly by a moment generated by the erector spinae muscles. Moments have to be calculated about a bending axis and this is taken to be in the lower lumbar spine, the position of this axis then defines a pivot about which the spine bends. As an extreme example the lower spine has even been described as being like a ball and socket joint (the spine) stabilised by tension guy wires (the muscles)[2]. Apart from the lack of anatomical realism in this approach, even in the early days of the model it was recognised that there were a number of potential problems. Among the first to become apparent was that the calculated forces were of the same magnitude as the failure strength of the vertebral bodies[3]. This was only slightly improved by invoking intra-abdominal pressure, acting between the soft tissues of the diaphragm and the pelvic floor, to provide an additional extensor moment. Though some more detailed models have reduced this[4] there is still little or nothing to spare between the calculated forces and the crushing strength of vertebrae. Other, similar, models still predict forces of over 3 tonnes in championship weight lifters[5], a factor of about three greater than the highest measured vertebral strengths. Related to this is the question of whether the spinal muscles are strong enough to generate the forces required[6]. This lead to the proposals of ligamentous and thoracolumbar fascia involvement to supplement the inadequate muscles[6,7], though it was subsequently shown that neither of the mechanisms proposed could work as suggested[8,9]. Careful measurements of muscle cross-sections suggest that more muscle may be available than first thought and with greater lever arms[10] and that this may be sufficient to provide the required moment. Even so, the whole system appears to be working close to physiological limits when lifting even modest weights. Another significant drawback with the lever model is that it concentrates on force calculation and takes little account of posture. The curved nature of the spine is considered more as a hindrance than a help and, consequently, is generally ignored. A simple angle of inclination from the vertical is typical of the only postural description used. This is clearly a gross oversimplification as weights that can be supported very easily in some postures are impossible in others[11].

A different approach to modelling the spine is to describe it as an arch-like structure[11-13]. Starting from the question, "How are forces transmitted through a curved structure?" leads to a model that relies on the curvature and flexibility of the spine to provide a stable, load-bearing structure. The closest analogy is an engineering arch, such as that found in a masonry bridge, which, if designed properly, is extremely stable under loads directed against the convex surface. These loads are balanced by a compressive force, or thrust, along the curve of the arch and there are no requirements for externally applied forces to provide stability. Most arches have their ends at the same height but this is not a necessity (flying buttresses for instance), provided the appropriate mathematical conditions for stability can be satisfied[12] an arch can be stable in any orientation. An analogy may be found by considering a string with weights hanging from it. This is stable (provided the string does not break) for a wide range of tensions in the string; the more taut the string is pulled the less the curvature. If now the string can be imagined to support compression and is inverted (Figure 1), it will still be stable as long as the compressive force applied to the ends is sufficient to balance the weights being applied and, by comparison, the smaller the curvature the greater the compression required for stability. This is the origin of the funicular polygon method of analysis[12].

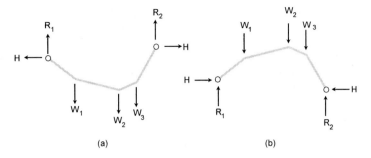

Figure 1. Analysing an arch is mathematically identical to analysing a string with weights hanging from it except that in (a) the string hangs and is in tension whereas in (b) the 'string' is now able to sustain compression and is inverted.

3. The arch model

Though still in its infancy, an arch-like description of the human spine appears to explain many of the experimental results which do not readily satisfy the predictions of the lever model. Among the principal predictions are considerably lower forces in the lumbar spine with a significant margin of safety compared with the failure strength of vertebrae. It reinterprets the functions of intra-abdominal pressure and the thoracolumbar fascia and provides an explanation for the complexity of the muscular anatomy. In addition, bounds can be placed on the static stability of the spine in terms of loads and postures which may be of considerable importance in ergonomic applications. Loads that are well within the capacity of an individual when they have freedom to choose the method of lifting may become excessive when the lifting method is constrained, for instance by a low roof in mining or the height of a bed for nurses lifting patients.

The principle difference between an arch and a lever is that an arch is a curved structure which, if constructed properly, is intrinsically stable whereas a lever needs to be externally supported. This stability is provided for an arch of a given geometry by generating compressive forces along its length, there is no requirement for externally applied moments to produce equilibrium. The way this works is easily demonstrated by considering a series of wooden blocks threaded onto a string (Figure 2). If the string is slack the blocks simply hang limply. However, the blocks can be made to project horizontally by holding the end block and pulling on the string. This now forms a structure which, clearly, is not stabilised by applying a bending moment. Stability is engendered by the compressive force generated along the line of bricks by the tension in the string. This analogy will be seen in the next section to be important when considering the role of the muscles and ligaments. Upper and lower bounds on the forces in an arch of a given shape can be calculated[12] and these are generally considerably less than for a cantilever as now there is no need for an externally applied balancing moment, the arch structure itself carries the load.

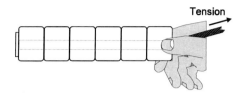

Figure 2. An unconnected series of blocks can be stabilised to form a structure by increasing the tension in the string passing through the centre. The string is an integral part of the structure and there is no externally applied bending moment.

Forces are considered to be transmitted through a structure along a trajectory called a thrust line. In general the actual thrust line in an arch structure is unknown but limits on those possible may be calculated from a knowledge of the shape of the arch and the applied forces. However, it is sufficient to find just one possible thrust line in equilibrium with all the forces and lying entirely within the depth of the arch ring to ensure that the arch is stable[12,14,15]. The nearer the thrust line lies to the centre-line of the arch then the greater the margin of safety for stability. It is not clear what constitutes the arch ring in the spine but a conservative approximation would be to limit it to the vertebral bodies. In practice, it may be that because of the load-bearing abilities of the apophyseal joints the effective depth is greater than this. The compressive thrust is generated along the whole length of the spine by muscles and ligaments attached to adjacent vertebrae or across several vertebrae. At any level in the spine, the component along the spine of any external force applied proximally and the sum of the forces from muscles and ligaments crossing that level all contribute to provide the necessary thrust[12].

A number of points arise immediately from this description of the spine. Firstly, the flatter the curvature of an arch the greater the axial force required to produce equilibrium. It is probably impossible to straighten the entire spine, there will always remain some curvature, but as the spine flexes from a standing posture, the lumbar spine starts to flatten and at about 30-40° of flexion the lumbar lordosis is starting to reverse its curvature[16,17]. The spine will then form a single slightly-curved structure. Because the curvature is small, postures that superficially may appear very similar may, in fact, give rise to markedly different forces[11]. The arch-like description is applicable to any posture the spine might adopt, whether it be doubly curved as in the normal upright posture, or almost flattened in flexion. It is also applicable to curvatures in three-dimensions such as found in scoliosis, though this has yet to be investigated. Fundamental to the arch concept is that predicting a possible thrust line within the structure determines whether it is stable or not and that it is possible to determine such a thrust line within any curved structure if the shape and loading are known. In this way the variations between the sexes as well as changes due to growth and ageing can all be analysed providing the shape of the spine is known, it is not sufficient simply to know the angles subtended by spinal segments.

4. Ligaments

The primary function of the spinal ligaments is mechanical, though they are innervated and may form part of a proprioceptive system. The innervation could also be nociceptive and be a cause of otherwise indeterminate back pain. However, little is known of either of these and only the mechanical function will be considered here. Ligaments consist of collagen fibres and, sometimes, some elastin embedded in a proteoglycan gel. Collagen fibres, like ropes, are only strong when placed in tension. In this way they can reinforce the weak gel if they are appropriately oriented within it and their orientations can be identified with the directions in which the tissue can sustain tensile forces[18]. Different combinations of similar components are used in all the soft connective tissues. By considering them as fibre-reinforced composite materials it is possible to estimate the interactions that are required to transfer stress to the fibres[19] and to show how reorientation of the fibres in a stretched ligament stiffens the tissue progressively[20]. The advantages conferred by this will become apparent. Though the spinal ligaments are generally thought to run the whole length of the spine the functions deduced from their structures are not all the same.

The anterior and posterior longitudinal ligaments and the ligamenta flava are to be found along the whole length of the spine. The collagen fibres have a preferred orientation parallel to the axis of the spine but the distribution of orientations is broad in the unstretched ligament and becomes more highly aligned as the ligament is stretched[20,21]. Thus the posterior longitudinal ligament and the ligamenta flava become stiffer as the spine is flexed and the anterior longitudinal ligament becomes stiffer as the spine is extended from its upright position[22-24]. They are prestrained in a spine from which the muscles have been removed by up to 10% for the anterior and 13% for the posterior longitudinal ligaments[21,23] as is shown by their retracting when cut. They are also viscoelastic which means that when loaded rapidly they are stiffer than when loads are applied slowly[21].

These longitudinally oriented ligaments will, therefore, maintain a compressive force along the axis of the spine throughout the whole range of flexion and extension. This thrust will help to stabilise the arch of the spine, as described above, and will help to prevent tensile forces developing which could potentially damage the outer fibres of the annulus fibrosus. These ligaments will increase the thrust as the spine flexes by an amount that depends on the speed of movement because of their viscoelasticity. Increasing the curvature of the spine will increase the force generated by the ligaments but will reduce the amount of force required along the arch for equilibrium. In this way the ligaments, which are stretched passively and do not themselves expend energy, will relieve the active muscles and thus reduce the muscular energy expended to hold a certain posture. The progressive stiffening of the ligaments at a rate which depends on the speed of stretching provides a mechanism for restricting not only the movement of the spine but also the rate of movement as the spine approaches the limits of its range of motion. If they were initially slack and tightened suddenly there would be a danger of their being snapped easily, and if their stiffness was constant they would not have the same braking effect and so damage to other tissues, such as the disc, might more easily result.

In contrast, the collagen fibres in the lumbar interspinous ligaments are oriented predominantly perpendicularly to the axis of the spine[25]. This is unlike how they are portrayed in text books, which normally depict the fibres oriented vertically, and suggests that they can provide little resistance to flexion of the spine. It has been shown that the interspinous ligaments are continuous with the thoracolumbar fascia[9] and therefore the main function of the ligaments appears to be to help anchor the thoracolumbar fascia to the spine. This supplements its insertions to the spinous processes and provides a continuous line of attachment. The fascia appears to have a complex function involving the dorsal muscles and intra-abdominal pressure, which will be discussed presently, and thus needs a strong attachment to the spine.

The supraspinous ligament similarly appears to have only a minor role in limiting extension of the spine[21]. It is largely loose, fatty tissue reinforced by a little collagen that is poorly oriented. No single, continuous longitudinal collagenous structure was found[21] and it is reported to terminate between L3 and L5 depending on the individual[26]. It is very weak when extended *in vitro* in an axial direction and it has been suggested that its primary function is to protect the spinous processes from traumatic injury. The spinous processes form the attachment surfaces for many spinal muscles and the thoracolumbar fascia and, as shown below, their loss or damage could conceivably affect the stability of the spine.

5. Muscles

5.1. Erector spinae

The number of muscle fascicles in the spine and the complexity of their organization commonly leads to their being approximated in any biomechanical modelling; for instance, by a single rope-like muscle running from the sacrum to the thorax. Recent careful dissection has revealed a very precise arrangement of muscle fibres in the lumbar erector spinae group of muscles[27] and in the lumbar multifidus[28]. The function of these muscles in the arch model of the spine has been discussed in detail previously[13], here I shall discuss some of the key ideas and show that the proposed function of something as commonplace as a muscle depends on the model into which it is being fitted.

Far from being a single muscle mass the lumbar erector spinae has been described in four distinct groups of muscle fibres[27]. It consists of two muscles, longissimus thoracis and iliocostalis lumborum, each with distinct thoracic and lumbar parts. There is a clear pattern to the insertions of the fascicles. Both the site of the insertion on each vertebra and the number of intervening vertebrae between the insertions are remarkably reproducible.

The thoracic fascicles of longissimus thoracis, termed longissimus thoracis pars thoracis, arise from the thoracic transverse processes and ribs and are inserted into the lumbar spinous processes, the sacrum and the ilium[27]. Those muscle fibres arising from T1 to T9 are inserted serially into the lumbar spinous processes from L1 to S4, *ie.* a separate muscle fascicle links T1 to L1, T2 to L2 etc. Those fascicles arising from T10 to T12 have insertions into the fourth sacral segment and rostrally along the posterior edge of the ilium between the posterior-inferior and posterior-superior iliac spines. These insertions mean that the muscle fibres run immediately adjacent to the vertebrae and consequently their distance from the bending axis is small. As the spine is flexed the muscle fibres will follow the curve of the spine and in all positions will lie immediately adjacent to the vertebral column. The lumbar part of longissimus thoracis, longissimus thoracis pars lumborum, consists of five fascicles lying lateral to the multifidus[27]. Each fascicle arises from the accessory and transverse processes of a lumbar vertebra and is inserted into the medial aspect of the posterior superior iliac spine. These attachments again mean that the muscle fascicles all lie close to the vertebral column. The bending moment they can apply is therefore limited by the short lever arm this confers. This was further demonstrated by Dumas *et al.*[29] who showed that the line of action of longissimus thoracis in the upright posture, taken as a whole, projected onto the sagittal plane is among the closest to the spinal axis of all the dorsal muscle groups.

Mechanically, a muscle fascicle such as those described can act only on *all* the vertebrae lying between its attachments. A muscle inserting between vertebrae T1 and L1, for instance, will not simply apply a force such as to extend T1. Vertebra L1 is not fixed and its position will be controlled by all the muscles which are attached to it. The force applied to T1 will be equal and opposite to that applied to L1 by the muscle fascicle being considered. For an arch-like structure, which requires a force to be developed around the curve of the arch, this is just the type of force which needs to be applied between two points to control the longitudinal stress and the bending moment in the structure. Because the thoracic spine is relatively inflexible[30] the part of the arch that needs most control is the flexible lumbar region. The longissimus thoracis pars thoracis, by its attachment to the lumbar vertebrae rather than directly to the sacrum, is well placed to be able to coordinate the control of the thoracic and lumbar regions of the spine. The fascicles of the lumbar part function in a similar way and are well placed close to the spinal axis to control the compressive forces within the lumbar curve.

The iliocostalis lumborum has also been described in two components, one attached rostrally to the thoracic vertebrae, the other to the lumbar vertebrae[27]. Iliocostalis lumborum pars thoracis arises from the dorsal aspect of the posterior superior iliac spine and the dorsal edge of the iliac crest and is inserted rostrally into the lower eight or nine ribs. Iliocostalis lumborum pars lumborum has its origins at the tips of the lumbar transverse processes and the middle layer of the adjacent thoracolumbar fascia of vertebrae L1 to L4 and is attached caudally to the ventral edge of the iliac crest. According to Macintosh and Bogduk[27] the lumbar fascicles constitute a considerable mass of muscle fibres connecting the tips of the lumbar transverse processes to the iliac crest and yet are largely unrecognised in textbooks. The iliocostalis lumborum forms the most posterior group of muscle fibres. It therefore has the largest lever arm with which to apply a bending moment to the spine. It is maximising this lever arm that is one of the key factors in the traditional lever model as this is crucial to it being able to generate the required extension moment to balance the flexion moment from weights being carried. However, in the arch model, though a bending moment is important, mechanical equilibrium is achieved through the compressive force along the spine. It would appear then that the bending moment produced by the iliocostalis has more to do with movement of the spine than with static equilibrium. Its line of action is such that it can control motion in the sagittal plane[29].

In the arch model it may be seen that the thoracic and lumbar components of the muscles not only have a common anatomy[27] but also a common mechanical function. This is in contrast to their proposed functions within the traditional lever model[31] in which the thoracic fascicles of both longissimus thoracis and iliocostalis lumborum are given separate functions to their lumbar parts. An arch-like structure also requires that the muscles must lie close to the axis of the spine. This is directly contradictory to the requirements of the lever model in which strenuous efforts have been made to maximise the distance from the vertebrae in order to increase the proposed lever arm of the muscles and hence reduce the demands on the force production of the muscles and the loads generated in the spine. So it can be seen that the ways in which muscle groups are believed to function are dependent on how the whole spine is modelled.

The flexibility of the spine and its curvature have other consequences. As the spine flexes and extends it does not maintain a rigid configuration. Movement is achieved by readjustment of the curvature, rather like bending a 'flexicurve'. Additional range of motion is obtained from rotation of the hips. The thoracic fascicles will extend the thoracic spine and have the effect of flattening the kyphosis while the lumbar components will control the positions of the lumbar vertebrae. The presence of a thoracic kyphosis means that some muscle fascicles will follow a curved path. This will result in the line of action of a muscle being deflected out of the straight line between its insertions and so effectively increasing the lever arm of the muscles. This means that muscles may generate larger moments in flexed postures than estimated simply from the anatomy of their attachments[4]. Concentration on a ball-and-socket-like spine has resulted in the neglect of where in the spine bending moments are applied by the muscles. For instance, a fascicle attaching L1 to the iliac crest cannot move this vertebra in isolation. The force it applies is not simply a bending moment about L5-S1, but it will have a bending effect about *all* the vertebrae which lie between its attachments and a component of compression along the spine. It will thus tend to increase the curvature of the whole lumbar region. The curvature of the spine, therefore, not only enables an arch-like structure to be developed but modifies the action of the muscles which have to be considered as an integral part of the structure.

5.2. Lumbar multifidus

The lumbar multifidus has been shown to consist of five separate bands, each arising from the spinous process and laminae of vertebrae L1 to L5[28]. Each band is innervated independently of all the others and contains fascicles that span two or more segmental levels caudal to it. For instance, the band from L1 has fascicles that pass caudally to the mammillary processes of L3 to S1 and a final fascicle that is inserted into the posterior superior iliac spine. The forces the lumbar multifidus can apply to the lumbar vertebrae have been analyzed by Macintosh and Bogduk[32] and shown to be primarily in the sagittal plane almost perpendicular to the spinous process and the pedicle. Being perpendicular to the lever arm of the spinous process ensures that the bending moment they can apply to it is at its most efficient[32]. With respect to an arch-like structure the lumbar multifidus is capable of controlling the local curvature of the lumbar spine. The separate innervation of each muscle band means that each vertebra is independently controllable and therefore the curvature of the lumbar spine can be adjusted very precisely to match the loading being imposed. It is the overall curvature, or posture, of the spine which determines its stability and therefore this control is necessary to its function as an arch-like structure.

5.3. Psoas major

The psoas major is usually known as a flexor of the hip[33], but in contrast to all other leg muscles it is attached proximally to the lumbar spine. Its anatomy and biomechanical action have recently been studied by Bogduk and colleagues[34] and it was shown to have little ability to flex or extend the spine. However, it was shown to exert considerable compressive and shear forces, both of which increase from L1-L2 down to L5-S1 segmental levels. The conclusion drawn was that psoas is intended to act on the hip and that the large compressive and shear forces was a price that had to be paid for a well-designed hip flexor[34]. However, fundamental to the arch hypothesis is that compressive forces are essential to the function of such a structure and that this is, in fact, the way in which stability and load bearing is achieved, not by having applied bending moments. In this context the psoas major appears to be ideally situated to help control the compressive and shear forces in the lower spine and possibly to coordinate the movement of the spine with the legs, which is a major factor in lifting heavy weights. This will be discussed in a later section.

6. Thoracolumbar fascia

The thoracolumbar fascia forms a tough sheath of connective tissue that surrounds the back muscles. The posterior layer is attached to the lumbar and thoracic spinous processes and the interspinous ligaments[9,35] and is comprised of two laminae; a superficial and a deep. The collagen fibres in the superficial lamina are oriented caudo-medially, at about $\pm 70°$ to the spinal axis, and those in the deep lamina are oriented caudo-laterally, at about $\pm 110°$ to the axis of the spine[9].

The belief that the spinal musculature was insufficiently strong to support loads with the spine flexed lead to various mechanisms being proposed for the thoracolumbar fascia to supplement the muscles. One proposal was that tension in the abdominal muscles, to which the thoracolumbar fascia is attached at its lateral margin, could apply an extensor moment to the spinous processes[7]. Measurement of the fibre orientations in the fascia[35] allowed the extensor moment to be calculated and it was shown to be only about 2% of the calculated extensor moment of the spinal muscles[8]. Another mechanism proposed was that additional tension in the fascia might be provided by the radial expansion of the back muscles as they contract. This was called the 'hydraulic amplifier' mechanism[36] and was thought to be able to generate an axial tension from the circumferential tension with a gain of about five. However it has recently been shown that the ratio of axial to circumferential tension is about 0.4[9]. So neither of these mechanisms can work as first thought.

The pattern of collagen fibre organisation in the thoracolumbar fascia is very similar to that found in the annulus fibrosus of intervertebral disc[37] which functions as a cylindrical pressure vessel[38]. As a muscle contracts along its length it expands radially. Constraining this expansion by a surrounding fascia applies a radially directed stress to the muscle and a theoretical analysis has suggested that this may increase the stiffness and the strength of the muscle, *ie.* for a given strain (axial contraction) it should be able to support a greater load than it would if it were unconstrained[39]. It has been estimated that this could increase the force in the spinal muscles by up to about 30%[40]. Though this mechanism would increase the efficiency of the spinal musculature it is not intended to address the problem of the supposed inadequacy of the back muscles. It is simply a consequence of constraining a material, in this case a muscle, when its dimensions are changing as loads are applied. The muscles appear to have adequate strength if loads are carried by the arch structure of the spine. Maybe more important are that increasing the axial stiffness of the muscles will increase their resistance to bending, and that the fascia will also constrain the muscles to lie along the curve of the spine. This latter will tend to reduce their lever arm but increase the compressive force they exert along the axis of the spine. Again this is what is required to stabilise an arch-like structure.

7. Intra-abdominal pressure

Intra-abdominal pressure rises during lifting manoeuvres and was invoked in the lever model to provide an additional extensor moment to try to reduce the problem of the large calculated muscle forces and lumbar stresses. However, rather than acting as a load reducing mechanism between the soft tissue structures of the diaphragm and the pelvic floor, not a very efficient use of pressure, it is proposed that it provides a compressive stress on the convex surface of the lumbar lordosis. The combined action of intra-abdominal pressure and the lumbar lordosis will increase the stress in the lumbar spine which in turn will have a stiffening effect on the structure[11-13]. This is especially important when lifting heavy weights where it has been noted that weight lifters could lift heavier weights if they maintained a lumbar lordosis than if they allowed the lordosis to straighten or reverse[41]. Though mechanical testing of individual motion segments show that they appear strongest when loaded in a position corresponding to a straight spine[42] the primary problem is not the strength of the spine but its stability. For this a lordotic posture is intrinsically more stable as it uses to the full the advantages inherent in an arch structure. The rapid rise and fall of intra-abdominal pressure at the start of a lifting manoeuvre means that its stabilising effect is greatest when it is most needed, *ie.* as the load is being accelerated. Reappraising the role of intra-abdominal pressure within the arch model of the spine provides solutions to some of the apparent anomalies in measurements of intra-abdominal pressure during various manoeuvres[43].

8. Stability of the spine

The curved, flexible spine forms an arch-like structure of which the muscles and ligaments are an integral part. Stable equilibrium of this structure is assured if suitable thrusts are generated along the curve of the arch to match the curvature and the applied loads. The ligaments and muscles cannot be considered as applying external forces but are, in fact, intrinsic to the structure. This is aptly demonstrated by studies of the isolated vertebral column, devoid of muscles, which collapses under axial loads of only about

2 kg^3. It is only the muscles that enable the spine to support considerable loads. However, rather than being like guy-ropes, the arch model suggests that they are an integral part of the structure. Tension in the muscles increases the compressive force along the spine and thereby increases its bending stiffness. This is a similar mechanism to that found in prestressed concrete beams in which tensioned steel bars along the centre of the beam increase the compressive stress in the beam and enable it to withstand considerably greater bending forces than if unstressed. Evidence for this mechanism in the spine can be found in studies in which compressive preloads on an isolated cadaveric spine were shown to decrease lumbar flexibility[44]. Several factors combine to generate this increased axial stress. Not only are the muscles tensioned but this will cause the lordosis to tend to flatten as a flatter arch is required to balance higher compressive forces. Intra-abdominal pressure, acting on the lumbar lordosis, may well increase and tension in the thoracolumbar fascia will stiffen the muscles. The net result is that the spine will straighten and its bending stiffness will increase. Recent results[45] suggest that this is exactly what happens when the spine is loaded *in vivo* by pure compression. Volunteers, standing erect, were given a weight to hold in each hand by their sides while muscular activity and length of the lumbar spine were monitored. As the weight carried was increased the spacing between markers on vertebrae S1 and T12 was found to increase and the lordosis decrease.

When considering forces in the lumbar spine, generally only the magnitude of the force is calculated. Forces, though, have a direction as well as a magnitude and forces generated in the spine have to be transmitted through the curved structure. For greatest stability, the vector sum of the applied forces, shown by the thrust line, should pass centrally along the axis of the spine and be perpendicular to each vertebra (Figure 3a).

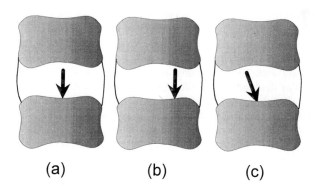

(a)   **(b)**   **(c)**

Figure 3. The magnitude, position and direction of the thrust line within the spine determine the normal force, bending moment and shear force respectively within the structure. (a) Shows a normal force, (b) also contains a bending moment and (c) a shear force but no bending moment.

If the thrust line remains normal to the vertebrae but passes at a distance from the midline it will apply a bending moment equal to the product of the force and the distance from the centre line (Figure 3b). A shear force will be generated only if the thrust line does not pass normally to the vertebra but is inclined at some angle (Figure 3c). An anteriorly directed shear is shown but this would clearly become posteriorly directed if the thrust line were to be angled to the right in the figure. This means that even at a segmental level that is markedly angled from the horizontal, such as L5-S1, there is only a shear force if the thrust line is not perpendicular to the sacrum. The role of the psoas now assumes a new importance as it is capable of generating a large anteriorly directed shear force which will be able to counteract those shear forces generated by the posterior muscles which must be posteriorly directed. Generation of a spondylolisthesis may not, therefore, simply be a result of fatigue due to the combination of body weight and a tilted vertebra, but could be a result of ill-judged manoeuvres causing the psoas to generate large unbalanced shear forces.

The dynamics of the spine has been little studied but one thing that is certainly true is that the spine does not pass through a series of equilibrium positions as it is extended from a flexed position, for instance when lifting a heavy weight from the floor. It has been reported that erector spinae electromyographic recordings were silent on starting to lift and that the spine only started to extend once the acceleration phase was over[30,46]. More detailed study is required to investigate how the weight is accelerated and the spine repositioned to enable the weight to be caught in an appropriate position to be held. However, as the spine is flexed or extended it will constantly adjust its curvature, it does not work like the jib of a crane by maintaining a fixed posture while the dorsal muscles raise or lower it. Similarly to the above description for static positions the curvature of the spine and the lumbar lordosis will increase the effectiveness of the dorsal muscles. It is worth noting that most anatomical studies only consider the positions of the muscles in an upright posture (the psoas muscle study above being a rare exception) and this provides little information on the line of action of the muscles in flexed postures when changes in the shape of the spine may considerably alter this. The thoracolumbar fascia constrains the radial expansion of the back muscles thereby increasing their strength and bending stiffness. Attachment of the fascia to the abdominal muscles will coordinate stress in the fascia with intra-abdominal pressure and together they will increase the bending stiffness of the lumbar spine during lifting manoeuvres.

The spine cannot be considered simply as a series of bones, discs and ligaments which is supported and moved by attaching a number of muscles and treating the assembly as a set of levers. In such a model, the number and complexity of the muscles and their innervation defy rational explanation, the calculated forces required for stability are dangerously large and no allowance is made for the curvature and flexibility of the spine. Instead it forms a complex, dynamic structure in which no part can properly be considered in isolation. The curvature of the spine makes it into a structure and, consequently, control of the curvature becomes essential. The muscles and ligaments then have to be considered as integral parts of that structure and their functions are carefully coordinated to maintain stability and control.

9. Acknowledgements

I wish to thank the Medical Research Council for a Senior Fellowship.

10. References

1. F.K. Bradford and R.J. Spurling, *The intervertebral disc* (Charles C. Thomas, Springfield, Illinois, 1945) p. 28.
2. Z. Ladin, K.R. Murthy and C.J. De Luca, *Spine* **14** (1989) 927.
3. J.M. Morris, D.B. Lucas and B. Bresler, *J.Bone Joint Surg.* **43-A** (1961) 327.
4. S.M. McGill and R.W. Norman, *Spine* **11** (1986) 666.
5. H. Granhed, R. Jonson and T.H. Hansson, *Spine* **12** (1987) 146.
6. S. Gracovetsky, H.F. Farfan and C. Lamy, *Spine* **6** (1981) 249.
7. S. Gracovetsky, H.F. Farfan and C. Helleur, *Spine* **10** (1985) 317.
8. J.E. Macintosh, N. Bogduk and S. Gracovetsky, *Clin.Biomech.* **2** (1987) 78.
9. K.M. Tesh, J. Shaw-Dunn and J.H. Evans, *Spine* **12** (1987) 501.
10. S.M. McGill, N. Patt and R.W. Norman, *J.Biomech.* **21** (1988) 329.
11. R.M. Aspden, *Appl.Ergonom.* **19** (1988) 319.
12. R.M. Aspden, *Spine* **14** (1989) 266.
13. R.M. Aspden, *Clin.Anat.* **5** (1992) 372.
14. J.E. Gordon, *Structures*, (Penguin Books Ltd., Harmondsworth, 1982) p. 171.
15. J. Heyman *The Masonry Arch*, (Ellis Horwood Ltd., Chichester, England, 1982)
16. H.F. Farfan, *Spine* **3** (1978) 336.
17. R. Cailliet, *Low Back Pain Syndrome*, (F.A. Davis Co., Philadelphia, 1980)
18. D.W.L. Hukins and R.M. Aspden, *Trends Biochem.Sci.* **10** (1985) 260.
19. R.M. Aspden, *Proc.R.Soc.Lond.* **258** (1994) 195
20. R.M. Aspden, *Proc.R.Soc.Lond.* **A406** (1986) 287.
21. D.W.L. Hukins, M.C. Kirby, T.A. Sikoryn, R.M. Aspden and A.J. Cox, *Spine* **15** (1990) 787.
22. A.L. Nachemson and J.H. Evans, *J.Biomech.* **1** (1968) 211.
23. H. Tkaczuk, *Acta Orthop. Scand. Suppl.* **115** (1968)
24. M.C. Kirby, T.A. Sikoryn, D.W.L. Hukins and R.M. Aspden, *J.Biomed.Eng.* **11** (1989) 192.
25. R.M. Aspden, N.H. Bornstein and D.W.L. Hukins, *J.Anat.* **155** (1987) 141.
26. P.M. Rissanen, *Acta Orthop. Scand. Suppl.* **46** (1960)
27. J.E. Macintosh and N. Bogduk, *Spine* **12** (1987) 658.
28. J.E. Macintosh, F. Valencia, N. Bogduk and R.R. Munro, *Clin.Biomech.* **1** (1986) 196.
29. G.A. Dumas, M.J. Poulin, B. Roy, M. Gagnon and M. Jovanovich, *Spine* **16** (1991) 293.
30. P.R. Davis, J.D.G. Troup and J.H. Burnard, *J.Anat.* **99** (1965) 13.

31.   S.M. McGill and R.W. Norman, *J.Biomech.* **20** (1987) 591.

32.   J.E. Macintosh and N. Bogduk, *Clin.Biomech.* **1** (1986) 205.

33.   P.L. Williams, R. Warwick, M. Dyson and L.H. Bannister *Gray's Anatomy*, 37th edn. (Churchill-Livingstone, Edinburgh, 1989)

34.   N. Bogduk, M. Pearcy and G. Hadfield, *Clin.Biomech.* **7** (1992) 109.

35.   N. Bogduk and J.E. Macintosh, *Spine* **9** (1984) 164.

36.   S. Gracovetsky, H.F. Farfan and C. Lamy, *Orthop.Clin.North Am.* **8** (1977) 135.

37.   W.G. Horton, *J.Bone Joint Surg.* **40-B** (1958) 552.

38.   D.S. Hickey and D.W.L. Hukins, *Spine* **5** (1980) 106.

39.   R.M. Aspden, *J.Mater.Sci.:Mater.Med.* **1** (1990) 100.

40.   D.W.L. Hukins, R.M. Aspden and D.S. Hickey, *Clin.Biomech.* **5** (1990) 30.

41.   R.W. Porter *Management of Back Pain*, (Churchill Livingstone, Edinburgh, 1986)

42.   W.C. Hutton and M.A. Adams, *Spine* **7** (1982) 586.

43.   R.M. Aspden, *Clin.Biomech.* **2** (1987) 168.

44.   J. Janevic, J.A. Ashton-Miller and A.B. Schultz, *J.Orthop.Res.* **9** (1991) 228.

45.   Parnianpour M, Patwardhan A and Aaron A. The effects of pure compressive load on the spine stability: a test of muscular coactivation. *Abstract from the International Society for Study of the Lumbar Spine Meeting, Heidelberg* (1991)

46.   W.F. Floyd and P.H.S. Silver, *J.Physiol.* **129** (1955) 184.

CHAPTER 2

FORCES ACTING ON THE LUMBAR SPINE

P. Dolan and M.A. Adams

1. Introduction

The importance of mechanical loading in the etiology of low back pain is widely accepted, and considerable efforts are currently being made to reduce spinal loading in the workplace. In some cases, however, these efforts may be misdirected because attempts to reduce one type of loading, for example compression, may lead to increased bending or torsional stresses on the spine. We need to understand all the components of mechanical loading before sensible steps can be taken to reduce them.

In the following sections we will consider compression, shear, torsion and bending. In each case, methods used to measure the component of loading will be described, and a brief account given of the magnitude of the loading to be expected during everyday activities. We will then consider specific factors, such as muscle fatigue, which can lead to increases in spinal loading. Finally, we will compare peak spinal loads *in vivo* with the forces known to damage the osteoligamentous lumbar spine *in vitro*, in order to give a realistic assessment of the dangers of back injury in the workplace.

2. Compressive loading

Most of the research into spinal loading has concentrated on assessing the compressive forces acting on the spine. These forces arise from a variety of different sources:

2.1. Superincumbent body-weight

The compressive loading on the lumbar spine due to superincumbent body weight is relatively small: approximately 55% of body weight, or 380 N for an average man[52]. (For comparison, 1 kg = 9.81 N - 'Newtons'.) However, body weight is effectively magnified when the body is accelerated because the inertial force is proportional to the acceleration. A fighter pilot might experience compressive forces up to about 10,000 N. when ejecting from a plane as a result of the high accelerations involved, and this is sufficient to fracture the vertebrae[29]. Similarly, a fall on the buttocks can involve a very rapid deceleration accompanied by a high impulsive compressive force, and *in-vitro* experiments suggest that the forces involved would be sufficient to cause burst fractures of the thoraco-lumbar vertebrae[21].

2.2. Muscle tension

During quiet standing and sitting, the compressive force on the lumbar discs is approximately 500 N and 700 N respectively[43]. Only 380 N of this is due to body weight, so the rest must come from the action of the back and abdominal muscles stabilising the upper body. During other activities such as bending forwards and lifting objects from the ground, the back muscles must generate large extensor moments (a 'moment' is a force multiplied by a distance). Because the erector spinae operate on short lever arms about the 'pivot point' in the centre of the intervertebral discs, they must generate very high tensile forces, and these act to compress the lumbar spine (Figure 1). During forward bending and lifting, compressive forces due to muscle tension can rise to 5 to 10 times superincumbent bodyweight[16,40].

2.3. Intra-abdominal pressure (IAP)

A pressurised abdomen probably reduces the compressive force on the spine by transmitting load directly from the shoulders to the pelvis. However, a raised IAP is normally associated with increased abdominal muscle activity, which would act to *increase* spinal compression, and so the true benefit of the IAP mechanism is hard to quantify. If a wide abdominal belt is used to help raise the IAP, then the compressive force on the spine may be reduced by about 15%[41].

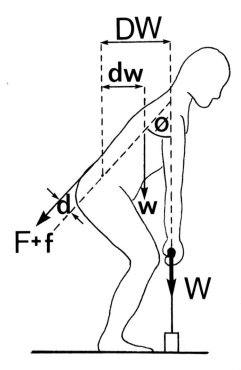

Figure 1. A simple model of forces acting on the lumbar spine when a person lifts a weight W. The total extensor moment (EM) is given by the following equation:

$$EM = W*DW + w*dw = (F+f)*d + M$$

where w is the weight of the upper body and arms, F the active tension in the back muscles, f the passive tension in muscles and fascia, and M the bending moment resisted by the osteoligamentous spine.

2.4. *Fascia, ligaments and passive tissue in muscles*

Tension in these structures can rise to levels sufficient to support the spine in full flexion. This is demonstrated by the fact that the back muscles fall electrically silent in flexed postures when they are said to exhibit 'flexion relaxation'[20]. During stoop and squat lifts of 10 kg, the lumbar spine is flexed by 96% and 83% respectively of its full range of movement between erect standing and full flexion, and under these circumstances, tension in the passive structures provides about 31% and 22% respectively of the total extensor moment required to lift the weight from the ground[19]. Calculations based on comparisons with cadaveric data suggest that most of this passive tension is generated in structures other than the intervertebral discs and ligaments, such as the lumbodorsal fascia and supraspinous ligament[19]. Using these structures during lifting is beneficial because they lie further from the 'pivot' than do the back muscles and intervertebral ligaments, and so impose a smaller compressive 'penalty' on the lumbar discs. Also, the energy stored in stretched passive tissues during a forward bending movement will be used to help the spine straighten-up with the weight[22]. Hence, oxygen consumption is reduced and lifting is less 'hard work'[33].

2.5. *Techniques for measuring the compressive force acting on the spine*

The 'gold standard' measurements are obtained by inserting a pressure-sensitive needle into a lumbar intervertebral disc[44]. Cadaveric experiments are required to calibrate the output of the pressure transducer against the compressive force acting on the spine[45]. Obviously, this method is too invasive for general use, and it may not be safe or accurate during vigorous movements. An alternative technique is to use movement analysis systems to measure the position, velocity and acceleration of each body segment. This data is combined with force-plate measurements of the ground reaction force, and input to a 'linked segment' model in order to calculate the compressive and shear forces acting on the lumbar spine[12,23,39]. The difficulty here is that large random errors are introduced when the raw (position) data is twice differentiated to give accelerations, which are required to compute forces. A third method of measuring compression makes full use of the fact that, during manual handling, most of the compressive force is generated by tension in the back muscles. The electromyographic (EMG) signal from these muscles can be calibrated against muscle tension generated during isometric contractions so that the EMG signal recorded during subsequent dynamic movements can be related to forces[16]. Corrections are necessary to account for changes in muscle length and the rate of muscle shortening[16]. This technique is only partially dynamic because it takes no account of axial accelerations acting down the spine. However, it does measure the forces associated with rapid angular accelerations of the spine which are not accurately computed by linked segment models. These can be considerable, as demonstrated in Figure 2, which shows how muscle activity and lumbar flexion vary during a 10 kg squat lift.

2.6. *Typical compressive forces acting on the lumbar spine*

These rise from 250 N, 500 N and 700 N respectively when lying supine, standing and sitting, to 1,900 N when holding a 5 kg weight in outstretched arms[43], and 5.5 kN when lifting a 30 kg weight from the ground[18,49].

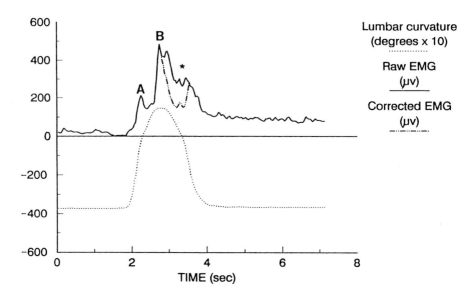

Figure 2. EMG activity of the erector spinae, and lumbar curvature, during a squat lift of 10 kg. At A, the back muscles slow the forward movement of the torso, and at B the weight is lifted from the ground. At B, the lumbar spine is flexed by approximately 52°. During the interval marked *, the lumbar spine is rapidly extending, so that the muscles are shortening. Under these circumstances, the EMG signal must be corrected for velocity effects before it can be compared with tension in the muscle.

3. Shear

The intervertebral shear force can be defined as the 'horizontal' force acting parallel to the mid-plane of the disc. This force has never been measured *in vivo*, but it is probably higher at the lowest lumbar levels where the discs are inclined at a steep angle to the horizontal, so that a substantial component acts to shear the joint. This component is increased in stooped postures, and when heavy weights are carried. One mathematical models suggests that it rises to approximately 760 N when a person marches with a heavy pack on the back[13]. However, other models based on detailed anatomical observations and EMG recordings suggest that the forward shear force can be limited to 200 N by the action of the lumbar back muscles pulling each vertebra backwards as well as downwards[50].

4. Bending

Until recently, very little was known about the bending stresses acting on the lumbar spine. Bending stress, or more correctly bending moment, increases markedly as the limit of lumbar flexion is approached. Recent work has shown that it is feasible to quantify the bending moment acting on the spine by measuring lumbar flexion *in vivo*, and then comparing the peak flexion angle with normalised bending-rotation curves determined in cadaver experiments on osteoligamentous lumbar spines[2]. Dynamic flexion angles are measured *in vivo* using the electromagnetic 3-Space Isotrak device (Polhemus) which can be attached to the skin surface overlying the spinous processes of L1 and S1. This technique has shown that people lifting weights from the ground commonly flex their spines by 80-95% of their range between upright standing and the fully flexed toe-touching position[18,19]. As a result, the peak bending moment on the spine during a squat lift of 10 kg rises to about 17% of its value at the elastic limit of the motion segment (when injury is first sustained[2]). This 17% corresponds to about 11 Nm on average, although this value almost doubles if a stoop lift is used[18]. Peak bending moments are also highly dependent on the size and weight of the load being lifted as well as its distance from the feet[18].

5. Torsion

The lumbar spine is subjected to torsional stresses during activities such as discus throwing. Also, there is a tendency for lateral bending movements to be 'coupled' with small torsional movements, although this effect appears to be variable and under muscle control[47]. In theory, it should be possible to measure torque *in vivo* by measuring axial rotation movements and comparing them with the torque-rotation properties of cadaveric spines. Unfortunately, the torque rises rapidly with angle of rotation[5] so that small experimental errors in the latter would entail large errors in the former. Skin movements lead to gross overestimates of axial rotation when measured by skin-surface devices such as the 3-Space Isotrak[46]. Accurate measurements of axial rotation can be obtained by inserting screws into the spinous processes[25,26,35] but this is invasive, and the movement patterns may well be influenced by pain. Consequently, practically nothing is known about the torque acting on the lumbar spine *in vivo*. Nevertheless, non-invasive measurements of axial rotation movements do give some indication of torsional stresses on the spine. These may be sufficient for occupational studies attempting to assess the risks of low back pain[37].

6. Factors which increase spinal loading *in vivo*

In-vitro experiments have shown that mechanical overload of the spine, particularly when it is caused by a combination of bending and compression, can damage the intervertebral discs and ligaments, and in some cases may cause intervertebral disc prolapse[6]. In life, the back muscles act to protect the spine by preventing excessive bending[7] but this protection is at the expense of increased spinal compression, as described in Figure 1. The back muscles are therefore responsible for optimising spinal loading to ensure that neither the bending nor compressive stresses rise to damaging levels. However, there are circumstances when the back muscles may not provide adequate protection to the underlying spine, and these will now be reviewed.

6.1. Lifting whilst bending forwards and to one side

Compared to lifting in the sagittal plane, this increases the bending moment on the lumbar spine by up to 30% on average[18] and localises tensile stress in the postero-lateral corner of the disc furthest from the axis of rotation. The component of lateral bending in this type of 'awkward' lifting is often assumed, incorrectly, to be torsion.

6.2. Bending and lifting in the early morning

After being unloaded overnight, the intervertebral discs swell up in tissue fluid and the spine is then very stiff in bending. In the lumbar spine the range of flexion is reduced by about 10% on average. During forward bending and lifting movements, the peak bending moment on the spine increases by 160% on average compared to later in the day[17].

6.3. Rapid and unco-ordinated movements

Large muscle forces are required to accelerate the upper body, and these increase during rapid movements. Lifting quickly can therefore cause the peak compressive forces on the spine to increase by between 20 and 100%[12,39,34,18]. This is demonstrated in Figure 3 which shows the effect of lifting speed on the bending and compressive stresses on the spine.

6.4. Poor lumbar mobility

The bending moment acting on the lumbar spine during lifting is inversely related to the range of lumbar flexion between erect standing and the extreme toe-touching position. Consequently, people with poor lumbar mobility consistently apply bending moments to their spines which are up to 100% higher than those observed in people with good mobility[15].

6.5. Fatigued back muscles

If the back muscles become fatigued they allow increased flexion of the spine during forward bending and lifting activities[51] (also, unpublished data from our own laboratory). Quadriceps fatigue is similarly associated with increased spinal flexion during lifting as subjects change from a predominantly 'bent leg' technique to a 'bent back' technique[54]. Such increases in spinal flexion could lead to increased strain in the intervertebral discs and ligaments.

6.6. Prolonged sitting and standing in flexed postures

Prolonged flexion causes creep stretching of ligaments and fascia[3,38] leaving a greater proportion of the overall bending moment to be resisted by the discs and muscles[3].

6.7. Exposure to vibration

Vibrations close to the 4-5 Hz natural frequency of the spine[55] cause large displacements and require considerable muscle tension in order to hold the upper body steady[53]. Hence, spinal compressive loading is increased. In addition, vibration exposure

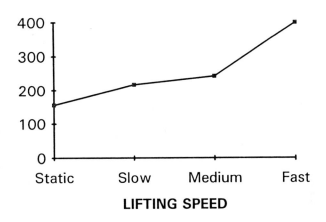

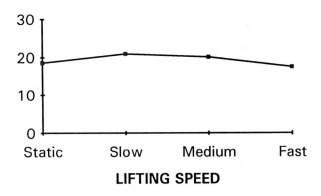

Figure 3. Spinal loading increases when weights are lifted rapidly. **Upper:** high angular accelerations of the trunk require high tensile forces in the back muscles, and this increases extensor moment (and spinal compression) by up to 100%. **Lower:** the bending moment acting on the osteoligamentous lumbar spine (expressed as a % of its value at the elastic limit) is little affected by speed of movement. (Data from Ref. 18.)

leads to fatigue in the erector spinae and external obliques[55] and this may reduce their ability to protect the spine, as discussed above. A further effect of vibrations may be to increase creep in the intervertebral discs, and this can lead to high concentrations of compressive stress in the annulus fibrosus[42].

The clinical significance of the above findings is supported by epidemiological studies which show that low back pain and acute disc prolapse are associated with repeated bending and lifting of heavy loads[32,37], sudden or unexpected loading[36] and long-distance driving[31].

7. Spinal loading required to cause injury

By comparing the mechanical strength of spinal tissues with the forces that act upon them *in vivo* we can obtain some indication of the possible mechanisms of spinal injury in everyday life. The ultimate compressive strength of male and female lumbar motion segments aged under 40 years is 7.8 kN on average[48]. However, repetitive loading over a few hundred cycles considerably weakens the motion segment causing many vertebrae to fail at about 50% of their ultimate strength[10,27]. People under 40 might therefore risk damaging their vertebrae during repetitive manual handling whenever the compressive force exceeds 4 kN. For older people, damage may occur at even lower loads because compressive strength falls with age[11]. The peak compressive force acting on the spine can be calculated, to a rough approximation, by dividing the peak extensor moment by the effective lever arm of the back muscles and fascia. If we assume that this lever arm is 7.5 cm for young male subjects[40] then the compressive force acting on the spine of such individuals rises from about 2.5 kN in a '0 kg' squat lift (picking up a pen) to 5.5 kN in a 30 kg lift[18]. Similarly, for 10 kg lifts, increasing the distance of the object from the feet from 0 cm to 60 cm increases the compressive force from 2.7 kN to 5.2 kN; and increasing the speed of lifting from 'medium' (4 s duration) to 'fast' (1 s) increases peak compression from 3.2 kN to 5.3 kN[18]. In each of these comparisons, a change in just one variable factor (speed, distance etc) was enough to raise the estimated compressive force above the 4 kN threshold for fatigue damage, so these factors can have a decisive effect on the risk of compressive injury to the vertebral body. Compressive forces may indirectly affect the discs also, since vertebral body damage can lead to abnormal stress concentrations in the adjacent annulus fibrosus[8].

The bending moment acting on the lumbar spine can affect the intervertebral discs and ligaments in a more direct manner. By definition, posterior ligament injury occurs when the peak bending moment during forward flexion reaches the elastic limit of the motion segment (100%), and fatigue failure of the discs can occur at this limit if the applied cyclic compressive force is approximately 3.5 kN[6]. In the series of experiments described above where different factors such as the size, weight and position of the load as well as the lifting technique were varied, we found that the average value of peak bending moment did not exceed 40% in any lift, suggesting that, during moderate lifts, the back muscles protect the underlying spine from excessive bending. However, bending moment can rise greatly in those individuals who have poor spinal mobility in the sagittal plane[15] and in such people the bending moment during lifting can often exceed 50% of that required to injure the motion segment in a single loading cycle. A relative load of 50% may be sufficient to cause fatigue failure if we assume that the discs and ligaments are weakened by repetitive loading to a similar extent as the vertebrae (see above). The risk of bending injuries is increased even further in the early morning because at this time of day, the intervertebral discs are still swollen with fluid after the night's recumbency. This increases their resistance to bending by approximately 300%[4]. Much of the effect is lost after the first hour of the day, but during this hour, the risk of bending injuries to the lumbar spine must be substantial.

The forward shearing force acting on the lower lumbar vertebrae can reach 760 N when marching with a heavy pack[13], but may be reduced to 200 N by muscle action[50]. The pars interarticularis will fail in a manner resembling spondylolysis when the shear force reaches about 2 kN[14]. A similar injury can result from repetitive loading at only 760 N[13], so it would appear that the intervertebral shear force could cause spondylolysis if the back muscles fail to resist it. Backwards bending of the inferior articular processes about the pars interarticularis is increased when the motion segment is loaded to simulate lumbar extension movements[24]. Conversely, full flexion movements generate high tensile forces in the apophyseal joint capsular ligaments, and these can bend the inferior facets forwards and down relative to the pars[24]. Thus, alternating full flexion and extension movements cause large stress *reversals* in the pars, and this may explain why sporting activities such as gymnastics and fast bowling (cricket) are closely associated with spondylolysis[28,30].

Outside the laboratory, manual handling tasks often combine several of the factors considered above. We suggest that their overall effect on the lumbar spine can be assessed by combining the results from more than one series of lifts. Thus, particularly high loading in bending and compression would occur during rapid reaching movements, during rapid stoop lifts, and when the object to be lifted is bulky, and awkwardly positioned relative to the lifter's feet. This may explain why epidemiological surveys show a close association between back injuries and sudden or awkward movements or postures[9,36].

A degree of uncertainty is inevitable when extrapolating from cadaveric material to living people because it is necessary to assume that each individual behaves like the average. This will give rise to random errors. However, systematic errors arising from changes in the spine's mechanical properties after death are likely to be small, as discussed in detail elsewhere[1]. Therefore, the comparisons made above between spinal loading *in vivo* and tissue strength *in vitro* are probably realistic and may serve to draw attention to particular aspects of spinal loading which may cause injury and subsequent back pain.

8. References

1. M.A. Adams *Spine* (1994) (in press).
2. M.A. Adams and P. Dolan, *J Biomech* **24** (1991) 117-126.
3. M.A. Adams and P. Dolan, *Clin Biomech* (1994) (in press).
4. M.A. Adams, P. Dolan and W.C. Hutton, *Spine* **12** (1987) 130-137.

5.   M.A. Adams and W.C. Hutton, *Spine* **6** (1981) 241-8.
6.   M.A. Adams and W.C. Hutton, *Spine* **10** (1985) 524-531.
7.   M.A. Adams and W.C. Hutton, *Clin Biomech* **1** (1986) 3-6.
8.   M.A. Adams, D.S. McNally, J. Wagstaff and A.E. Goodship, *Eur Spine J* **1** (1993) 214-221.
9.   M. Bovenzi and A. Zadini, *Spine* **17** (1992) 1048-59.
10.   P. Brinckmann, M. Biggemann and D. Hilweg, *Clin Biomech* **3** **(Supplement 1)** (1988).
11.   P. Brinckmann, M. Biggemann and D. Hilweg, *Clin Biomech* **4** **(Supplement 2)** (1989).
12.   M. Buseck, O.D. Schipplein, G.B.J. Andersson and T.P. Andriacchi, *Spine* **13** (1988) 918-21.
13.   B.M. Cyron and W.C. Hutton, *J Bone Joint Surg* **60-B** (1978) 234-8.
14.   B.M. Cyron, W.C. Hutton and J.D.G. Troup, *J Bone Joint Surg* **58-B** (1976) 462-466.
15.   P. Dolan and M.A. Adams, *Clin Biomech* **8** (1993) 185-192.
16.   P. Dolan and M.A. Adams, *J Biomech* **26** (1993) 513-22.
17.   P. Dolan, E. Benjamin and M.A. Adams, *J Bone Joint Surg* **75B Supp I** (1993) p22.
18.   P. Dolan, M. Earley and M.A. Adams, *J Biomech* **27** (1994) 1237-1248.
19.   P. Dolan, A.F. Mannion and M.A. Adams, *J Biomech* **27** (1994) 1077-1085.
20.   W.F. Floyd and P.H.S. Silver, *J Physiol* **129** (1955) 184-203.
21.   B.E. Fredrickson, W.T. Edwards, W. Rauschning, J.C. Bayley and H.A. Yuan, *Spine* **17** 9 (1992) 1012-21.
22.   S. Gracovetsky and H. Farfan, *Spine* **11** (1986) 543-571.
23.   K.P. Granata and W.S. Marras, *J Biomech* **26** (1993) 1429-38.
24.   T.P. Green, J.C. Allvey and M.A. Adams, *Spine* **19** (1994) (in press).
25.   G.G. Gregersen and D.B. Lucas, *J Bone Joint Surg* **49-A** (1967) 247-262.
26.   R. Gunzburg, W. Hutton and R. Fraser, *Spine* **16 (1)** (1991) 22-29.
27.   T.H. Hansson, T. Keller and D. Spengler, *J Orthop Res* **5** 4 (1987) 479-87.
28.   P. Hardcastle, P. Annear, D.H. Foster, T.M. Chakera, C. McCormick, M. Khangure and A. Burnett, *J Bone Joint Surg* **74(B)** No3 (1992) 421-425
29.   C. Hirsch and A. Nachemson, *Acta Orthop Scand* **31** (1961) 135-45.
30.   D.W. Jackson, L.L. Wiltse and R.J. Cirincone, *Clin Orthop* **117** (1976) 68-73
31.   J.L. Kelsey *et al*, *Spine* **9** (1984) 608-13.
32.   J.L. Kelsey, P.B. Githens, A.A. White and T.R. Holford *et al*, *J Orthop Res* **2** (1984) 61-66.
33.   S. Kumar, *Ergonomics* **27** (1984) 425-433.
34.   T.P.J. Leskinen, *Ergonomics* **28** (1985) 289-291.
35.   R.M. Lumsden and J.M. Morris, *J Bone Joint Surg* **50-A** (1968) 1591-1602.
36.   A. Magora, *Scandinavian Journal of Rehabilitation Medicine* **5** (1973) 186-190.
37.   W.S. Marras, S.A. Lavender and S.E. Leurgans *et al*, *Spine* **18** (1993) 617-28.

38.   S.M. McGill and S. Brown, *Clin Biomech* **7** (1992) 43-46.
39.   S.M. McGill and R.W. Norman, *J Biomech* **18** (1985) 877-885.
40.   S.M. McGill and R.W. Norman, *J Biomech* **20** (1987) 591-600.
41.   S.M. McGill and R.W. Norman, M.T. Sharratt, *Ergonomics* **33** (1990) 147-160.
42.   D.S. McNally and M.A.Adams, *Spine* **17** (1992) 66-73.
43.   A. Nachemson, *Spine* **6** (1981) 93-97.
44.   A. Nachemson and J.M. Morris, *J Bone Joint Surg* **46A** (1964) 1077-1092.
45.   A.L. Nachemson, *Acta Orthop Scand* **(supplement 43)** (1960).
46.   M.J. Pearcy, *Spine* **18** 1 (1993) 114-9.
47.   M.J. Pearcy and S.B. Tibrewal, *Spine* **9** (1984) 582-7.
48.   O. Perey, *Acta Orthop Scand* **(supplement 25)** (1957).
49.   J.R. Potvin, S.M. McGill and R.W. Norman, *Spine* **16** 9 (1991) 1099-1108.
50.   J.R. Potvin, R.W. Norman and S.M. McGill, *Clin Biomech* **6** (1991) 88-96.
51.   J.R. Potvin and R.W. Norman, Can fatigue compromise lifting safety? Proceedings of the Second North American Congress of Biomechanics, Chicago, August 1992.
52.   S. Ruff, Brief acceleration: less than one second. In: German Aviation Medicine, World War II, Washington D.C., U.S. Government Printing Office 1: (1950) pp.584-597.
53.   R.E. Seroussi, D.G. Wilder and M.H. Pope, *J Biomech* **22** (1989) 219-229.
54.   J.H. Trafimow, O.D. Schipplein, G.J. Novak and G.B.J. Andersson, *Spine* **18** (1993) 364-7.
55.   D.G. Wilder, B.B. Woodworth, J.W. Frymoyer and M.H. Pope, *Spine* **7** (1982) 243-54.

CHAPTER 3

WHAT IS LUMBAR INSTABILITY?

D.W.L. Hukins

1. Introduction

A Medline search reveals that 23 scientific papers were published on spinal instability in 1992; in the same year, Nachemson wrote that "no scientific evidence exists on how to make the diagnosis of lumbar instability"[1]. Perhaps the term "instability" should never have been introduced. However, for better or for worse, patients are diagnosed as having lumbar instability and the term continues to appear in the literature. Under the circumstances, I believe it is worthwhile to explore what is meant by it.

I shall begin this chapter with a brief review of the literature. This review is not intended to be comprehensive but merely serves as a background to what follows. I then describe what has become the conventional biomechanical view of instability and what I believe to be its shortcomings. I shall then discuss the concept of stability from the standpoint of control theory and, finally, consider how this can be applied to the lumbar spine.

2. Background

A paper by Kirkaldy-Willis and Farfan[2] is frequently cited as a source of information on instability. However, their paper presents two completely different definitions of the term. One is that instability is "the clinical status of the patient with back problems who with the least provocation steps from the mildly symptomatic to the severe episode". The other is that it is "abnormal increased deformation with stress". This second definition is closest to what most authors mean by instability. It also has the advantage that, at least in principle, it could be diagnosed in a clinical examination. Such an examination would involve determining if abnormal motion were associated with some defined task. Unfortunately, however, the emphasis in the paper by Kirkaldy-Willis and Farfan is on the first definition which is based on a retrospective view of the history of an individual's pain once it has become severe. They show that the sudden onset of severe pain has certain similarities with the appearance of discontinuities in behaviour which are predicted by catastrophe theory. However, since back pain is a multi-factorial problem[3], it is difficult to see how a single cause for the onset of severe pain could be identified in an individual. Therefore, although their study is of fundamental interest, it is likely to be of little diagnostic value and it is mainly concerned with a view of instability which is substantially different from the usual one.

Nelson has given a more practical account of instability which he defines as the "intermittent mechanical failure of the spinal unit under load"[4]. This definition is very close to the second given by Kirkaldy-Willis and Farfan, i.e. it coincides with the usual view of the problem. He goes on to write that "the clinical picture depends on the underlying cause and is characterized by low back pain related to activity and relieved by rest". This statement could make the definition very broad. In principle, each cause could lead to different clinical signs, yet each set of signs would still be considered as instability. However, this potential problem is overcome when his list of underlying causes is considered. They are:

- spondylosis or disc degeneration
- spondylolisthesis
- trauma
- infection
- spinal tumours
- previous extensive surgical decompression.

Clearly, degeneration, trauma and surgical removal of parts of its structure can alter the mechanical properties of the spine to the extent that it does not function properly. The mechanical function of the spine also depends on the integrity of its alternating column of intervertebral discs and vertebrae. If the former are disrupted by infection or the latter by a tumour, the mechanical function will be impaired. These causes are all consistent with impaired mechanical integrity of the spine.

Spondylolisthesis demonstrates this impaired mechanical integrity very clearly, to the extent that "spondylolisthesis" and "instability" are often considered to be synonymous. However, although spondylolisthesis is a common cause of "intermittent failure", the list above shows that it is not the only one. In an erect posture, the weight, W, of the body acts vertically along the axis of the spine and so tends to compress it. The spine is able to withstand this compressive load because of the properties of the discs and the vertebral bodies. Bone tissue is stiff in compression because its mineral component causes it to resemble a ceramic[5]. The disc can withstand compression because its internal swelling pressure allows it to support a load, in much the same way as the pneumatic pressure in a tyre supports the weight of a vehicle. However, the ability of the disc to function in this way is highly dependent on its structure[6-7]. The list above shows that degeneration, trauma and pathology can all impair mechanical function. Figure 1 shows how the body weight affects the lumbar spine in flexion. The body weight, W, still acts vertically downwards but this direction no longer coincides with the axis of the spine. Now the compressive load is reduced to $W \cos \alpha$, where the axis of the spine is inclined at an angle, α, to the vertical direction. More importantly, a component $W \sin \alpha$ tends to shear the upper vertebra anteriorly, with respect to the lower vertebra. In the healthy spine this tendency to shear is resisted by tension in the posterior elements of the spine and the annulus fibrosus of the disc, as well as by the action of muscles tending to compress the disc, as described in Chapter 1. For example, shear tends to stretch the capsules of the zygoapophyseal (facet) joints and the posterior annulus fibrosus. Because both these tissues are stiff, they cannot stretch very much and so prevent shear[8]. However, trauma to the vertebral arch, tearing of posterior soft tissues, pathological changes etc. can all impair the resistance to shear. If this occurs, the upper vertebra may slip forward during flexion, under the action of the component $W \sin \alpha$, i.e. spondylolisthesis occurs[9]. A similar posterior shift during extension, retrolisthesis, may be observed if anterior tissues are damaged. The importance of tension of the posterior elements in preventing spondylolisthesis may explain the success of artificial ligaments

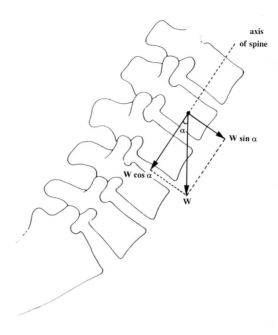

Figure 1. Spondylolisthesis under the action of the weight, W, of the body which always acts vertically downwards. The body is flexed so that its weight acts at an angle, α to the spinal axis. The compressive component of the weight is W cos α and a component W sin α tends to shear the upper vertebra anteriorly.

connecting the vertebral arches in preventing some forms of back pain as described in Chapter 19.

The problem of instability usually manifests itself when rising from a flexed posture. The patient demonstrates jerky movement, called an "extension catch", and may require the assistance of the hands and arms to resume an erect posture[10]. Although there tends to be a consensus on the importance of this observation, the circumstances surrounding it are not so clear in the literature. Kircaldy-Willis and Farfan state that, "The patient is not able to reach forward because of pain and on return to an erect position after forward bending, a catch in the back can be seen"[2]. Porter states that, "The patient frequently exhibits an exceptionally good range of forward flexion. The normal smooth motion of the spine is broken by a sudden broken movement, the extension catch"[10]. In the circumstances it seems fair to conclude that there is "no general agreement on the definition, the pathology or the clinical manifestation of lumbar instability" but that it manifests itself as "unnatural movement at one or more intervertebral levels"[10].

3. Biomechanical model

Pope and Panjabi considered a stable spine to be one which was in equilibrium under the action of the forces to which it was subjected[11]. They used the behaviour of a cone resting on a horizontal surface to illustrate the properties of a body in equilibrium. Figure 2 is based on a diagram in their paper and shows the three types of equilibrium for the cone. These types of equilibrium depend on how the cone behaves when it is displaced. If the cone is pushed from its position of stable equilibrium (resting on its base) it will return to its original position, provided it is not pushed too hard. This behaviour is the starting point for their mechanical view of stability and is in contrast to the behaviour of a body in neutral or unstable equilibrium. The displaced position of a body in neutral equilibrium is a new equilibrium position. For example, pushing a cone which is lying on its side simply rolls it to a new rest position. When a body in unstable equilibrium is displaced, it moves until it reaches a completely different equilibrium position. This behaviour is exemplified by a cone which is balancing on its tip; the slightest displacement causes it to fall on to its side, i.e. it moves from a position of unstable equilibrium to a position of neutral equilibrium.

In their paper, Pope and Panjabi equated stability with stable equilibrium but recognised an important difference between the spine and the simple model of Figure 2. Both tensile and compressive forces are involved in maintaining the spine in an equilibrium position. The vertebral bodies are joined by the outer lamellae of the annulus of the disc and the vertebrae are further tethered by a system of ligaments. An applied force which tends to displace one vertebra with respect to another tends to stretch these soft tissues. The fractional increase in their length is termed "strain". Because they are stiff, it is difficult to induce high strains in these tissues and so they resist the movement. When the tissues are strained in this way, they are in tension and will contract to their original length when the applied force is removed, i.e. they act rather like springs. Thus the system is in equilibrium under the action of an applied force because it is balanced by the tensile force in the strained tissues. Denoting the strain by ϵ, and the stiffness by E (measured in N m^{-2} or Pa), this tensile force (measured in N) is given by

$$F = \epsilon EA \qquad (1)$$

where A is the cross-sectional area of the tissue (in m^2), perpendicular to the direction in which it is strained. A simple example of how a tensile force resists an applied force is provided by a dog's lead - pulling back the dog when it pulls but otherwise exerting no force.

Figure 3 shows how a system can be maintained in stable equilibrium under the action of both tensile and compressive forces. In this figure the cone is balanced on its tip but is in stable equilibrium because it is tethered by three guy ropes. The tension in these guy ropes returns the cone to its original position when it is displaced. A compressive force is also involved in Figure 3 because the cone is being squashed against the horizontal surface. Similarly, when the spine is in equilibrium the vertebral column is in compression while its ligaments are in tension. Thus the system of Figure 3 provides simple model which illustrates the principles involved in maintaining the spine in stable equilibrium.

Pope and Panjabi then used the principles exemplified by Figure 3 to explore the conditions which led to stable equilibrium[11]. They noted that the stiffer the guy ropes, in this figure, the more difficult it would be to displace the cone. Equating stability with stable equilibrium they concluded that "stability [is] affected by the stiffness of the restraints". Therefore, they concluded, "instability is loss of stiffness". There is no doubt that a spine which could flop around, like an inverted cone with slack guy ropes, would not be in stable equilibrium. This model has subsequently been refined by Panjabi[12-13]. He proposes that a spine in equilibrium has a region of laxity around its equilibrium position which he calls the "neutral zone". The range of this neutral zone can be increased by injury and possibly by degeneration. This led Panjabi to a rather more complicated definition of instability[13]. "Clinical instability is defined as a significant decrease in the capacity of the stabilizing system of the spine to maintain the intervertebral neutral zones within the physiological limits so that there is no neurological dysfunction, no major deformity, and no incapacitating pain." In developing this concept, Panjabi also noted the importance of the musculature in generating active tension when required to maintain stability[12]. The importance of muscles for maintaining stability had been noted earlier[14] and will be developed further in this chapter.

The problem with equating stability with equilibrium is that it neglects the most important mechanical function of the spine - its flexibility. The spine is not a static system and so does not remain in equilibrium under the action of the forces to which it is subjected. Instead, it twists and bends to a variety of positions which may be adopted as static postures or, instantaneously, during locomotion. During at least some stages of movement the body cannot be in equilibrium because a system which is in equilibrium does not move, by definition. The stability of a moving system cannot be analysed as if it were static. For example, when running, the position of the centre of gravity of the body tends to make the runner fall forward. An analysis of the forces acting on the body when it is in this position would show that it is not in equilibrium. However, there is no sense in which this posture is unstable because it is a natural part of running and so is an integral part of effective locomotion. In the previous section, it was shown that instability of the lumbar spine is associated with movement. Indeed, the literature suggests that jerky movement, associated with returning from a flexed to an upright stance, is one of the few uncontentious signs of instability. The next section describes the control and stability of dynamic systems of this kind.

4. Control theory

Control of a dynamic system will be illustrated by the simple case of movement from an initial point, whose position is given by $x = 0$, to a final point, whose position is given by $x = 1$. However, the theory involved is not restricted to simple mechanical systems. A body changes its state of motion when a force acts on it. In biological systems, movement is initiated by a force, or pattern of forces, generated by muscular contraction. The resultant force need not be constant but can depend on time, t, and so

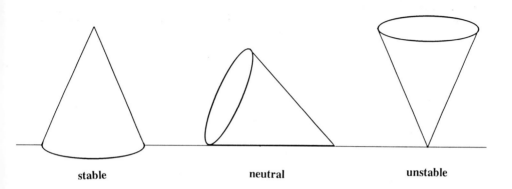

stable   **neutral**   **unstable**

Figure 2. Stable, neutral and unstable equilibrium illustrated by a cone resting on a horizontal surface.

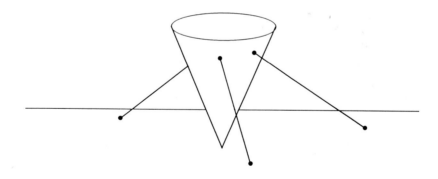

Figure 3. Tensile forces in three guy ropes can convert unstable equilibrium of a cone resting on its tip to stable equilibrium.

may be written as $F(t)$. The changes in x which arise from the application of this time-dependent force can be determined by solving an equation of the form of Eqn. 2. Readers who wish to skip the rest of this paragraph should still be able to follow the arguments that follow subsequently but will have to take more on trust. The behaviour of a second-order control system, which includes a mechanical system like the spine, can be described[15] by a differential equation of the form

$$a_0 x + a_1 (dx/dt) + a_2 (d^2 x/dt^2) = F(t) \qquad (2)$$

where dx/dt represents the rate of change of x (velocity) and $d^2 x/dt^2$ is the rate of change of velocity (acceleration). The bold face denotes that $F(t)$ and x are vectors (as are velocity and acceleration which are functions of x), i.e. that the direction of x is determined by the direction of $F(t)$. Here position is defined by the length of x which is denoted by x. The coefficients a_0, a_1 and a_2 in Eqn. 2 are a measure of the stiffness, energy dissipation (friction or viscosity) and inertia (mass for linear motion, moment of inertia for rotational motion) of the system, respectively. (Note that a_0 in Eqn. 2 is proportional to E in Eqn. 1). For movement of the spine, the coefficients a_0, a_1 and a_2 are functions of x, i.e. the system is non-linear. The reason that a_0 and a_1 are not constant is that the properties of the tissues of an intervertebral joint depend on how much it is compressed, twisted or bent. The value of a_2 changes because movement of the spine changes its shape and, therefore, its moment of inertia. Unfortunately, for a non-linear system, Eqn. 2 must be solved numerically which requires values for the coefficients over the ranges of motion to be considered. In this chapter the properties of a control system will be illustrated by the properties of a one-dimensional linear second-order system; Eqn. 2 can then be solved analytically[15]. The justification for this approach is that it illustrates the essential features of the control and stability of a mechanical system and that any non-linear system approximates to a linear system for sufficiently small changes in x. In this section we consider a system which is initially at rest with $x = 0$; at an instant in time, defined by $t = 0$, $F(t)$ changes its value so that the system moves towards a new state characterised by $x = 1$. The form of the solution of Eqn. 2 then depends on the value of a damping factor defined by

$$\zeta = (a_1^2 / 4 a_0 a_2)^{1/2} \qquad (3)$$

The behaviour of the system also depends on the value of its natural frequency

$$\nu_0 = (1/2\pi)(a_0/a_2)^{1/2} \qquad (4)$$

In the absence of any energy dissipation, i.e. when $a_1 = 0$, the system would continue to oscillate with this frequency indefinitely. Thus energy dissipation is responsible for damping the motion of the system. This result is important for understanding shock-absorption in the spine as well as for this chapter[16]. The way in which the value of ν_0 affects the behaviour of the system can be allowed for simply by plotting x against

$$\tau = 2\pi\nu_0 t \tag{5}$$

instead of plotting x against t.

Figure 4 shows how the system responds to instantaneous application of a force which tends to move it from an initial position of $x = 0$ to a final position of $x = 1$. Notice that the system does not immediately move to its final position. The way in which it moves depends on the value of the damping factor, ζ, defined in Eqn. 3. When $\zeta = 1$, the system is said to be "critically damped" and moves steadily from its initial to its final position. When $\zeta > 1$, the system is "over damped"; in this case the final position may not be attained in a reasonable time (note that τ in Figure 4 is a measure of time and is defined in Eqn. 5).

The system of Figure 4 shows the jerky behaviour characteristic of the extension catch when $\zeta < 1$. Instead of showing the smooth movement of the critically damped system, it now behaves in the manner which is characteristic of lumbar instability. However, in control theory a system is only considered to be unstable if it continues to oscillate and never reaches a rest position[15], as shown in Figure 5. The unstable spine shows oscillatory (jerky) behaviour but does finally come to rest with the required posture. Therefore, the unstable spine may not show "instability" in the sense in which the term is used in control theory. This does not matter if the theory aids our understanding of spinal instability. Furthermore, the patient with an unstable spine may push against the arms of a chair or the front of the thighs to return from a flexed to an upright posture[10]. Thus he or she is modifying the system in order to assist in the effort to reach the required position. In the absence of this extra assistance, it may not be possible to reach this position and so the body might then behave more like the system of Figure 5.

If the signs of lumbar instability arise from a reduction in the value of the damping factor, ζ, the question which then arises is what changes in the spine lead to this reduction? In principle the value of ζ can be reduced for three reasons:
•in the increasing stiffness, i.e. an increase value of a_0.
•increasing inertia, i.e. an increase in the value of a_2,
•decreasing energy dissipation (reduced damping), i.e. a decrease in the value of a_1,
The implications of this result will be discussed in the next section.

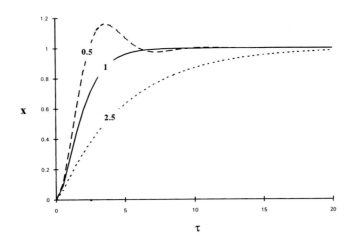

Figure 4. Behaviour of a simple control system in which the damping factor, ζ, has values of 1 (critically damped), 2.5 (over damped), and 0.5 (under damped). In this figure the displacement, x, is plotted against a variable, τ, which is related to time by Eqn. 5. At a time defined by τ = 0, a force is applied to move the system from its initial position, given by x = 0, to a final position given by x = 1.

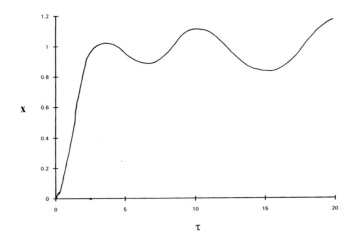

Figure 5. Behaviour of a simple control system, like that in Figure 4, which is truly unstable. It continues to oscillate and never tends towards a final position, in contrast to the behaviour exemplified by Figure 4.

5. Application to the spine

The first conclusion to be drawn from the previous section is that reduced stiffness cannot lead to the jerky movement which is characteristic of lumbar instability. This conclusion contrasts with the view of Pope and Panjabi[11] who believed that "instability is loss of stiffness" (see Section 3). However, there is little doubt that lack of stiffness in the posterior elements can be responsible for spondylolisthesis. Spondylolisthesis is considered to be a cause of instability and the two terms are often considered to be synonymous (see Section 3). Thus spondylolisthesis and the jerky movement associated with extension catch appear to have different causes. Whether reduced stiffness is considered a cause of instability depends on whether it is defined in terms of spondylolisthesis or jerky movement. Of course, some patients may have spondylolisthesis and exhibit the extension catch, but this does not mean that the two have a common cause.

An increased body mass will increase inertia and, hence, may lead to the onset of jerky motion. It would be interesting to determine whether patients who exhibit jerky movement have a significantly higher body mass than other chronic low back pain patients. Perhaps these patients should be encouraged to lose weight, in order to regain better control of their movement. During bending, the inertia of the body also depends on the length of the spine - the greater the length the greater the inertia. (This follows from the definition of moment of inertia). Thus it is predicted that taller patients are more likely to exhibit jerky movement than shorter patients.

However, it is reduced energy dissipation, i.e. inadequate damping, which is the most obvious cause of jerky movement. Energy is dissipated during movement of the spine because of the viscoelasticity of its component tissues and because of fluid flow. For example, compression of the spine leads to gradual expression of fluid from the intervertebral disc. Some of the energy involved in compressing the spine is then used to initiate fluid flow and cannot be recovered, i.e. fluid flow provides an energy dissipation mechanism. It may be that fluid flow is implicated in the viscoelastic response of tissues like ligament; if this were the only energy dissipation mechanism a better description of the behaviour of these tissues would be "poroelastic" but it is also likely that they exhibit intrinsic viscoelasticity[17]. Whatever the underlying mechanism, the tissues of the spine can dissipate energy. However, energy dissipation takes a finite time so that little energy can be dissipated during rapid movement. The example of fluid flow can be used to illustrate the way in which energy dissipation depends on time. It takes a finite time to squeeze fluid through the pores of a tissue, so that energy cannot be dissipated more rapidly than fluid can be squeezed out. Passive mechanisms, such as fluid flow and viscoelasticity may then be too slow to accomplish effective damping during movement. For example, the shortest time constant (relaxation time) associated with compression of the spine is about 20 min[18].

Muscles can also contribute to damping. Connective tissues, like ligaments and disc, dissipate energy in response to the forces to which they are subjected, i.e. their response to movement is passive. In contrast, muscles are able to apply forces to modify movement under the control of the nervous system. These forces are not simply a passive response to an applied force but arise from a conscious or reflex decision to generate force. This force is generated actively by chemical changes within the muscle cell and not by passive recoil. Contraction of antagonist muscles, which oppose movement, then provide a mechanism for adaptive control[19]. The effect of this adaptive control is to provide negative feedback which increases the value of a_1 in Eqn. 2, thus preventing the excessive movement which leads to the oscillatory behaviour when $\zeta < 1$ (see Figure 4). This adaptive control is feasible because the frequencies associated with nervous transmission are high compared with those associated with movement[20].

Therefore, stability of the spine involves both the nervous and the musculoskeletal system. Jerky movements associated with instability could then arise from a deficit in either of the two. Indeed, the causes of instability may differ from one patient to another and could prove very difficult to determine. As a result it appears sensible to define lumbar instability in terms of simple observable signs. The information summarised in Section 2 suggests that lumbar instability could then be defined simply as "unnatural movement". This definition could be preceded by the adjective "painful" but this is probably unnecessary because nobody complains of a condition which does not cause pain.

6. Acknowledgements

I thank Professor R.W. Porter for introducing me to the problem of lumbar instability and Mr G.F.G. Findlay for inviting me to give a lecture on spinal instability, at the Ninth Liverpool Spine Course, on which this Chapter is based. I am also grateful to Drs R.M. Aspden and S. Lees for useful discussions on control theory and stability.

7. References

1.   A.L. Nachemson, *Neurosur. Clin. N. Amer.*, **2** (1991) 785.
2.   W.H. Kirkaldy-Willis and H. F. Farfan, *Clin. Orthop.* **516** (1982) 110.
3.   G. Waddell, in *The Lumbar Spine and Back Pain*,3rd edn., ed. M. I. V. Jayson (Churchill Livingstone, Edinburgh, 1987).
4.   M.A. Nelson, in *The Lumbar Spine and Back Pain*,3rd edn., ed. M. I. V. Jayson (Churchill Livingstone, Edinburgh, 1987).
5.   D.W.L. Hukins, in *The Lumbar Spine and Back Pain*,3rd edn., ed. M. I. V. Jayson (Churchill Livingstone, Edinburgh, 1987).
6.   D.W.L. Hukins, in *The Biology of the Intervertebral Disc*, vol. 1, ed. P. Ghosh, (CRC Press, Boca Raton, 1988).
7.   D.W.L. Hukins, *Proc. Roy. Soc. Lond.* **B249** (1992) 281.
8.   M.H. Berkson, A. L. Nachemson and A. B. Schultz, *J. Biomech. Eng.* **101** (1979) 53.
9.   I.W. McCall, in *The Lumbar Spine and Back Pain*,3rd edn., ed. M. I. V. Jayson (Churchill Livingstone, Edinburgh, 1987).
10.   R.W. Porter, *Management of Back Pain* (Churchill Livingstone, Edinburgh, 1986).

11.   M.H. Pope and M. Panjabi, *Spine*, **10** (1985) 255.
12.   M. Panjabi, *J. Spinal Disorders*, **5** (1992) 383.
13.   M. Panjabi, *J. Spinal Disorders*, **5** (1992) 390.
14.   D.W.L. Hukins, in Back Pain: *Classification of Symptoms*, eds. J. C. T. Fairbank and P. B. Pynsent (Manchester University Press, Manchester, 1990).
15.   M. Healey, *Principles of Automatic Control* (Hodder and Stoughton, London, 1975).
16.   J.E. Smeathers, *Eng. Med.* **13** (1984) 83.
17.   D.W.L. Hukins, in *Connective Tissue Matrix*, part 2, ed. D. W. L. Hukins (Macmillan, London, 1990).
18.   A.D. Holmes and D. W. L. Hukins, *Med. Eng. Phys.* submitted.
19.   N. Hogan, *IEEE Trans. Autom. Control,* **29** (1984) 681.
20.   D.W.L. Hukins, in *Concise Encyclopaedia on Biological and Biomedical Measurement Systems*, ed. P. A. Payne (Pergamon, Oxford, 1991).

CHAPTER 4

TOWARDS A LOGICAL BASIS FOR THE DESIGN OF SPINAL IMPLANTS

J. Dove

1. Introduction

The Stoke-on-Trent Spinal Service began in 1980 with the appointment of the author to a busy orthopaedic unit with the facilities of a bio-engineering laboratory with a long track record in association with orthopaedic surgery. Since that time the broad spinal research programme has been under the heading of "the practical biomechanics of the internal fixation of the spine". Within this area there have been two main objectives; the development of the Hartshill system for the internal fixation of the spine and a pure research programme directed towards the *in vivo* measurement of the forces sustained by spinal implants in order to provide a logical basis for the future design.

2. The development of the Hartshill system for the internal fixation of the spine

The Hartshill system is a development from the Luque system for the segmental posterior internal fixation of the spine[1]. Initially the system consisted purely of a range of lengths of rectangles secured to the spine by segmental sublaminar wires. The first rectangle was implanted in January 1983. Over the years since then based on a programme of clinical studies together with biomechanical testing there have been a number of modifications and improvements to the Hartshill system.

2.1. The rectangles
Initially the rectangles were made only from stainless steel rods of a calibre of 5 mm. The range has now been extended to include 6 mm calibre rectangles primarily for spinal deformity and thoracolumbar fractures and 4 mm calibre rectangles for use in the cervical spine.

2.2. The wires
We have carried out extensive biomechanical studies on the wires appropriate for sublaminar fixation[2-4]. There are now three categories of wire which are colour coded; yellow tipped wire (0.86 - 0.914 mm diameter wire) for general use, red tipped wire (1.16 -1.219 mm diameter wire) for use where the forces are higher particularly in spinal deformity, thoracolumbar fractures and at the upper end of the lumbar rectangles and white wires (0.86 - 0.914 mm diameter wire) for use in the cervical spine.

2.3. The Ransford loop
A loop-shaped modification has been developed for occipito cervical fixation[5].

2.4. Pedicle screw bridge

This modification has been developed to allow a standard rectangle to be secured to a standard AO cancellous screw in a lumbar pedicle[6]. Pedicle screw bridges for use in the cervical spine have also been developed[7].

2.5. The Hartshill horseshoe

This device has been developed for use at the front of the lumbar spine to supplement an anterior disc excision and fusion. The first device was implanted in July 1988 and following a period of thorough biomechanical testing and clinical trials at two centres was five years later released for general use[8].

Twelve years on the results of our first consecutive 1000 rectangles with a minimum two year follow have been assessed and clinical results for a variety of spinal disorders have been reported both from our own and other centres: low back pain[9,10], spinal deformity[11-13], spinal fractures[14,15], spinal tumours[16] and cervical spine disorders[17,18].

3. Towards a logical basis for the design of spinal implants

Historically the design of spinal implants has been on a purely empirical basis. An implant of what was thought to be appropriate size was developed and if it failed it was arbitrarily strengthened. Little was carried out in the way of biomechanical testing. Much of what testing there has been made use of animal spines; in particular calf spines. We have shown that one has to be very wary of drawing conclusions about the loads in human spines from the results of calf spine studies[19].

The essential problem in the appropriate design of the spinal implant is that the forces to which that implant will be subjected in the long term are not known. Little has been done in the past to measure *in vivo* the forces to which spinal implants are subjected. The first studies involved measuring at surgery the forces to which Harrington rods were subjected in spinal deformity correction[20,21]. The same unit went on to conduct a pioneering study in scoliosis patients[22]. At that time it was the practice in that unit following surgical scoliosis correction with a Harrington rod to reoperate a fortnight later in order further to distract the curve. In four patients at the initial surgery Harrington rods with strain gauges applied were implanted and for two weeks following the surgery it was possible by a telemetry system to monitor the loads to which the rods were subjected.

We decided to develop this work further with a view to being able to monitor the forces over a longer period.

3.1. Strain gauge application

Much of the technology regarding strain gauges is standard. For much of the *in-vivo* work modification of standard pacemaker technology is suitable. There is little difficulty in laboratory conditions in applying strain gauges to a Hartshill rectangle and then measuring the loads whilst the implant is subjected to fatigue testing in a simple rig. In relation to *in-vivo* work however there is a major problem in finding a fixative which will both tolerate *in-vivo* conditions for a suitable period and be biocompatible. We carried out extensive studies using a large range of different fixatives to apply strain gauges to Hartshill rectangles that were fatigue tested in a bath of saline at body temperature[23-25]. Eventually a complex method of bonding the strain gauges to the rectangles was achieved so that the suitable signals could continue to be obtained for up to 120 days[26].

3.2. Animal studies

Having developed a suitable laboratory technique for the bonding of the strain gauges to the rectangles the next step was to perform animal studies. In the first instance we used sheep but they proved to be an unsatisfactory model for studies involving sublaminar wiring[27]. Investigation suggested that the baboon might be a suitable model. A telemetry system with a number of novel features was developed[26]. A strain-gauged Hartshill rectangle was then implanted in a baboon and very satisfactory signals were recorded for 38 days prior to sacrifice[24].

4. The future

Now that it has been shown that suitable recordings over a reasonable period can be obtained *in vivo* from a spinal implant the plan is to extend the experiment to human studies. First further animal studies further to improve the strain gauge and telemetry system are required. We then intend to conduct human experiments initially involving patients in whom it would anyway for clinical reasons be the intention to remove the spinal implant at a later stage.

It is hoped that this research programme will eventually result in our being able to record over an acceptable period the forces to which spinal implants are subjected thus providing a logical basis for their future design.

5. References

1.   E.R. Luque, ed. *Segmental Spinal Instrumentation*. Slack 1984.

2.   R.J. Crawford, P.J. Sell, M.S. Ali and J. Dove, *J Bone Joint Surg* **71-B** (1989) 151.

3.   N.R. Boeree and J. Dove, *J. Bone Joint Surg.* **74-B Supp 1** (1991) 91.

4.   N.R. Boeree and J. Dove, *Spine* **18** (1993) 497.

5.   A.O.Ransford, H.A. Crockard, J.L. Pozo, N.O. Thomas and I.W. Nelson, *J. Bone Joint Surg.* **66-B** (1986) 173.

6.   A.T. Rahmatalla, G.W. Hastings, J. Dove and A.H. Crawshaw, *Biomedical Engineering* **13** (1991) 97.

7.   J. Dove, *European Cervical Spine Research Society*, Rome (1994).

8.   N.R. Boeree, N. Valentine and J. Dove, *Proceedings Soc. Back Pain Research* (1991) 88.

9.   J. Dove, *Clinical Orthopaedics* **203** (1986) 135.

10.   E. Frish, M.D. Hoyle and J. Dove, *International Society for the Study of the Lumbar Spine*, 1988.

11.   J. Dove, *Orthopaedics* **10** (1987) 955.
12.   M. Onimus, *Revue d'Orthopedie* **1** (1987) 268.
13.   N. Valentine and J. Dove, *Combined meeting Scol. Res. Soc. Eur. Sp. Deformity Soc. Amsterdam*, 1989.
14.   J. Dove, *Injury* **20** (1989) 139.
15.   J. Bejui, M.H. Fessey, G. Anania and B. Tramond, *Lyon Chir.* **87** (1991) 150.
16.   C.S.B. Galasko, *J. Bone Joint Surg.* **73-B** (1991) 104.
17.   J. Dove, in *Cervical Spine II*, ed. R. Louis and A. Weidner, (Springer-Verlag, 1989) 79.
18.   G. Malcolm, A.O. Ransford and H.A. Crockard, *J. Bone Joint Surg.* **76-B** (1994) 357.
19.   J. Dove, R. Chan, K. Davis and M.S. Ali, *Scoliosis Res. Soc.*, Burmuda 1986.
20.   T.R. Waugh, *Acta Orthop. Scandinavica* (1966) 93.
21.   C. Hirsch and T.R. Waugh, *Acta Orthop. Scandinavica* **39** (1968) 136.
22.   A. Nachemson and G. Elstrom, *J. Bone Joint Surg.* **53-A** (1971) 445.
23.   P.J. Sell and A.H. Crashaw, *Strain* (1988) 21.
24.   P.J. Sell, *The development of a radio-telemetry system for the measurement of load and surface strain on a spinal implant*. M.Sc.thesis, Keele University, 1990.
25.   A.H. Crawshaw, *Securing reliable strain telemetry data on the Hartshill rectangle implant in vivo*. M.Phil. thesis, North Staffordshire Polytechnic 1992.
26.   P.J. Sell and J. Dove, *Proc. Inst. Mech. Eng.* (1989) 69.
27.   R.J. Crawford, *An investigation into the biomechanics of segmental spinal instrumentation using in vivo measurement*. MS thesis. Bristol University, 1991.

CHAPTER 5

BIOMECHANICS OF THE INTERVERTEBRAL DISC - DISC PRESSURE MEASUREMENTS AND SIGNIFICANCE

D.S. McNally

1. Introduction

The intervertebral disc has the important mechanical role of transmitting large loads whilst providing the spine with flexibility. Clearly to understand the function and dysfunction of discs, the internal as well as the external mechanical behaviour of the disc must be known. In order to investigate the internal mechanical environment of the disc measurements of stress and strain within the disc tissues themselves must be measured. This article describes techniques to measure such stresses, and illustrates the significance of the measurements.

1.1. A brief history of disc pressure measurement

The development of disc pressure measurement has closely followed the development of pressure measurement technology. The earlier measurements used a fluid filled catheter to couple the pressure within the disc to an external transducer. A simple mechanical system of a mercury filled line coupling the pressure to a Bourdon gauge was first used[1]. Later strain gauge electrical transducers were developed and were coupled to the nucleus using static and perfused saline filled catheters[2,3]. The use of fluid filled lines as a coupling medium have three major disadvantages:

a. The nucleus pulposus has a high osmotic potential which is much greater than that of the physiological saline normally used to perfuse catheters. This may cause the transducer system to under-read.

b. Compliance of the catheter or transducer may cause the intrusion of disc material into the coupling catheter at high pressures[2]. If the disc material is sufficiently solid it may occlude the catheter causing it to under-read.

c. The intact intervertebral disc has a very small compliance[3], hence perfused systems will cause large measurement artefacts.

Several attempts have been made to overcome these difficulties, whilst still keeping the basic liquid-coupled system

a. Silicone oil has been used to eliminate osmotic interactions between the coupling medium and the disc tissues[4].

b. The compliance of the transducer system has been reduced by removal of air bubbles using a vacuum chamber[4].

c. The measurement system can be pre-pressurised so that it is approximately the same as that of the disc[5]. This minimises fluid flow along the coupling catheter, but only provides a coarse estimate of disc pressure.

d. The coupling liquid can be separated from the disc tissues by a membrane[2]. This membrane also attenuates the pressure transmitted to the transducer so that a conventional blood pressure transducer can be used. This attenuation is dependent upon the mechanical properties of the membrane and the compliance of the coupling system. Since the system is now sealed and relatively non-compliant it is also temperature sensitive.

More recently miniature transducers have been developed which can be mounted on the end[6,7], or side[8] of a needle or catheter. The remainder of this article discusses the use of such side mounted transducers.

It is important to realise that strain gauged membrane pressure transducers do not measure pressure. They simply quantify the deformation of the membrane. In a well designed transducer the recorded deformation is that resulting from forces acting normally to the membrane (they are usually comparatively insensitive to shear). Such a transducer therefore records the component of stress acting normally to the transducer membrane. This is quite different to liquid perfused systems which record hydrostatic pressure in the liquid at the end of the catheter.

1.2. Stress profilometry

The simultaneous measurement of stress with position is common in the field of urology. Normally the procedure is to draw a transducer mounted on the end/side of a catheter through the urethra (although fluid perfused systems are also used)[9]. This technique is now standard and has been fully validated[10].

It is possible to apply this urological technique for the measurement of compressive stress within soft tissues to intervertebral disc mechanics. This gives a much more detailed insight into the internal function of the intervertebral disc than the snap shots of the centre of the nucleus previously described.

2. Stress profile measurement

The basic equipment required to make stress profile measurements comprises a stress transducer and a device to identify the position of the transducer within the disc. The system developed at Bristol is described below.

2.1. Stress transducer

The stress transducer[8] mounted on a 1.3 mm diameter needle is shown in Figure 1. The transducer element itself consists of a 3.0 mm x 1.2 mm x 0.1 mm beryllium copper plate. The central 2.0 mm x 0.8 mm region has been electrochemically etched to form a diaphragm 30 μm thick. Two thin film chromium cermet strain gauge elements were deposited onto the membrane and connected to form a half bridge.

The transducer element was fitted into a specially machined cut-out on the side of a 1.3 mm diameter stainless steel needle. The element was supported with epoxy formers and sealed with silicone elastomer. This construction has established a transducer system which is sufficiently robust to withstand repeated withdrawal from loaded intervertebral discs. The current experimental life time of a transducer seems to be of the order of one year of continuous use.

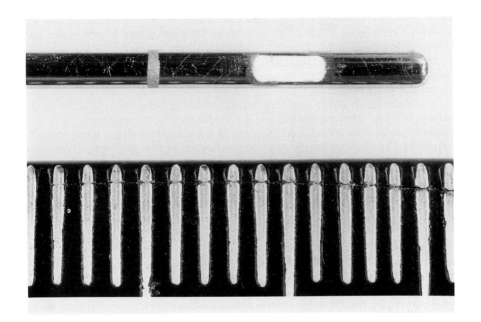

Figure 1. Photograph of the stress transducer (the white rectar   ) mounted on the side of a 1.3 mm diameter needle. The scale divisions are 1.0 mm.

2.2. Positioning system

In common with many urological profilometry systems the transducer is drawn through the disc at a constant speed, the position of the transducer therefore corresponds to a time. The transducer is pulled through the disc using a crystal controlled stepping motor[11]. This ensures that speed stability was better then 0.01 %. For most profile work a speed of 3.75 mm s^{-1} has been chosen, although the measurement was not speed dependent[11].

2.3. Profilometry technique

Although the stress transducer is designed to withstand very high distributed stresses it can be damaged quite easily by the application of bending moments and point loads. It is important to take care when inserting the transducer to prevent damage.

A cannula is normally used to introduce the transducer. This is inserted, over a 1.3 mm diameter hypodermic needle, equidistant from the two endplates (normally along a diameter of the disc). The hypodermic needle is the withdrawn and the transducer needle inserted through the cannula. The canula is then withdrawn over the transducer needle. This mechanism ensures insertion of the needle with minimal damage to the disc or transducer.

Stress profiles are taken by using the stepper motor to draw the needle through the disc at a constant speed. Throughout the profile the needle is supported to prevent the application of bending moments to the transducer needle since these can lead to measurement artefacts.

Normally two stress profiles are recorded, one with the transducer membrane parallel to the endplates (the vertical profile) and one with the needle rotated through 90°. This allows two orthogonal components of compressive stress to be recorded.

2.4. Features of a stress profile

Stress profiles show much variation both between individuals and between levels. However there are a number of features which are common to most profiles. A pair of stress profiles, illustrating common features of such measurements, is shown in Fig. 2.

Normally there is a central region of a pair of profiles where the stress is uniform and isotropic[11]. The isotropy indicates that the disc material is behaving as a fluid (not supporting shear stress) in this region. The uniformity suggests that the fibres in the disc matrix are not under tension. Isotropic compressive stress with no shear stress is effectively a hydrostatic pressure. Hence it is valid to quote a pressure at the centre of most discs. A point to note is that this region frequently extends into parts of the disc which behave a fibrous appearance[11,12]. This illustrates the danger of making inferences about the mechanical behaviour of disc tissues based purely upon their appearance.

At both edges of the disc there are regions where the compressive stress falls off rapidly with distance. It is these regions where the pressurised nucleus is retained by tensile stresses in the fibres of the annulus. It is possible to calculate the tensile loading of the from the gradient of the compressive stress curves using an analytical model[12].

Frequently there are concentrations of compressive stress in the disc matrix in one or more annular regions. These concentrations are usually anisotropic and therefore suggest that these regions are supporting shear stress and are therefore behaving more as a solid.

Finally some discs (such as the one in Figure 2) exhibit areas of inner annulus/nucleus where the stress is neither uniform nor isotropic. Again these regions are behaving more as a solid rather than the hydrostatic centre.

To conclude, stress profilometry enables the internal mechanical environment of the intervertebral disc to be investigated and quantified. Some of this behaviour is quite different to that which is normally assumed, and is often not in line with the appearance of the disc.

3. Internal intervertebral disc mechanics

The internal mechanics of intervertebral discs is affected by a large number of internal and external factors. This makes stress profiles very variable in appearance both between subjects and between level, and also with load and load history within a level. It also means that the technique is very useful for determining the changes in disc mechanics which are due to often quite subtle changes in external conditions.

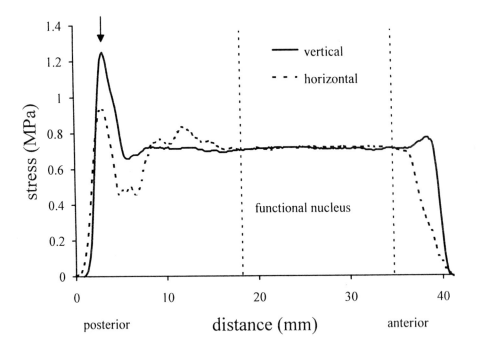

Figure 2. A stress profile of a disc under 1000 N pure compressive load showing a uniform, hydrostatic functional nucleus, a stress concentration in the posterior annulus (marked by arrow), and anisotropic non-uniform stress between the posterior stress concentration and the functional nucleus.

3.1. The significance of stress concentrations

A common feature of stress profiles are concentrations of stress in one or other annulus such as the one marked with an arrow in Figure 2. As will be discussed later these concentrations seem to have significant connections with ageing, degeneration and damage, they move about with changes in posture and seem to predispose disc prolapse.

A stress concentration is characterised by a peak in the stress profile localised in a region of annulus. The stress at the concentration is not normally isotropic, hence the disc is probably under shear at this point. Shear forces acting on a gel-like substance are normally very damaging and can lead to fracture and fissuring.

A simplistic view of this behaviour is to think of disc material being forced down the gradient of a concentration. At the peak of the concentration the disc material is forced apart down both slopes, so that the annulus is in effect tearing itself apart.

Another point to consider when thinking about concentrations of compressive stress in the annulus is that this stress will be transmitted to the adjacent vertebral endplate. Therefore, a concentration corresponds to focal loading of the endplates. Such loading may therefore not only be damaging to the disc, but also to the vertebrae.

3.2. Age and degeneration

Differences in the internal distribution of stress with age and degeneration have been observed[11]. Since age and degeneration are linked, its is hard to separate their effects.

Young non-degenerate discs have very large functional nuclei (regions of uniform isotropic stress) which extend to within approximately 4 mm of the edge of the disc. The compressive stress then falls off very rapidly with distance towards the edge, indicating that the load is transferred to tensile forces in the fibres of the annulus[12].

As discs get older and more degenerate the functional nucleus becomes smaller[11]. A larger proportion of the annulus seems to be recruited to take tensile loading. As degeneration becomes more severe the incidence of stress concentrations in the annulus increases. The disc in these areas is therefore behaving as a solid, rather than a liquid or a membrane in tension.

3.3. Posture

The overall loading of the disc, as well as the internal distribution of load, is dependant upon the angle of flexion of the vertebra/disc/vertebra unit. This is partly because flexion of the spine stretches the intervertebral ligaments resulting in a greater load being placed upon the segment at large flexion angles[11,13]. In extension the disc is loaded less due to increased loading of the facet joints[2,11,14]. Similarly the magnitude of a compressive preload affects disc height and therefore ligament tension, this leads to changes in the loading of the disc with flexion angle[15]. However, for small deviations in flexion angle from the neutral position the loading of the disc due to extra-discal structures has been shown, using disc stress measurements, to be minimal[11,13].

The effects of posture on intervertebral disc stress profiles have been studied in an experiment using 16 cadaveric intervertebral discs[13]. When loaded at 2000 N concentrations of stress (a maximum stress in the annulus of at least 110% of the mean stress in the functional nucleus) were found in the posterior annulus of 12 of the 16 discs. At 75% of the elastic limit of flexion of the segment, these concentrations were absent in 9 of the 12 affected discs, but concentrations were now observed in the anterior annulus of 3 of the discs. Peak loads in the posterior annulus were also found to significantly decrease under 75% of the elastic limit of flexion. There was no evidence to suggest that mean load on the functional nucleus changed over this range, suggesting that the intervertebral ligaments were not putting an additional load on the disc at 75% of the elastic limit of flexion. This is direct evidence to suggest that flexion of intervertebral discs changes the balance of loading, frequently removing stress concentrations from the posterior annulus.

3.4. Damage

Damage to the disc or endplate (or nucleotomy, or even prolonged creep loading) normally result in a loss of material from the nucleus, either by prolapse or by dehydration, resorption etc.. Since in all these cases can be thought of as loss of nuclear material it is not surprising that they have a similar effect on stress profiles to one another.

It has been demonstrated[16] that removal of disc material leads to a reduction in intradiscal pressure. This of course poses the question as to which structures are additionally loaded to produce this load relief from the nucleus. Loss of nuclear material normally results in a decrease in disc height and this loss can lead to additional loading of the facet joints, however this is not the whole story.

Minor compressive damage to the vertebral endplate, resulting in approximately 1.3 mm of disc height can affect the distribution of load across the disc itself[17]. The effect of this damage on the stress profiles is highly dependant upon the amount of flexion or extension applied to the disc, and also the age of the specimen.

In the experiment described above the damage generally resulted in a lowering of stress in most regions of the disc. This might be expected since a 1.3 mm loss of disc height is known to cause significant loading of the facet joints[18]. However, there was little evidence to suggest a similar reduction in peak stress in the posterior annulus. In fact, in specimens aged more than 50 years, there were found to be significant increases in the incidence of stress concentrations in the posterior annulus.

Stress profilometry therefore provides evidence which indicates that loss of nuclear material not only changes the loading of the disc by additional loading of other structures, but also that the distribution of stress within the disc is altered. Further this redistribution gives rise to concentrations of stress within the posterior annulus which might give rise to further damage.

3.5. Predisposition to prolapse

The previous illustrations of the use of stress profilometry have shown how it can be used to increase our understanding of the effects of degeneration or injury. In this final example it will demonstrated that the internal mechanical behaviour of the disc can also be used to predict its susceptibility to damage.

Intervertebral disc prolapse has been induced *in-vitro* by using a combination of high compressive loads and hyperflexion[19,20]. An interesting observation from these studies is that not every disc will prolapse under these conditions, more frequently the vertebral endplates fracture. There would therefore seem to be a predisposition to prolapse in some discs.

Stress profilometry was used to determine whether a predisposition to prolapse arose from a feature of the internal mechanical behaviour of certain discs[21]. Twenty-two intervertebral discs were loaded to destruction following stress profile measurements with the disc loaded in both in its neutral position and in flexion (similar to, but not as extreme as that subsequently employed by the destructive loading).

In 10 of the 22 cases the annulus failed but in 12 the failure was in the vertebral endplate. This reinforces the concept that there is some mechanical feature which predisposes prolapse.

There was no evidence to support the hypothesis that the magnitude of the loads in the disc were related to their failure mode. This suggests that prolapse is not due to simple overloading of the annulus. The important finding was that it was the presence and greater relative magnitude of stress concentrations in the posterior annulus when the disc was loaded in flexion which corresponded to failure of the posterior annulus.

These results suggest that the presence and relative magnitude of stress concentrations in the posterior annulus (rather than the over loading of the annulus) under sub-failure loading can be used to predict prolapse under more severe loading. Since stress concentrations seem to be regions of the annulus under a damaging stress regime, this identifies progressive internal mechanical damage of the intervertebral discs as a possible cause of disc prolapse.

4. New directions

Stress profilometry has already increased our understanding of the internal mechanics of intervertebral discs. Simply the measurement of the distribution of compressive stress has allowed mathematical models of the disc to be improved[12,22]. There is still a great deal of room for the further modelling of the more unexpected features of the stress profiles such as the stress concentrations.

Currently most stress profilometry has been carried out by pulling the transducer through the centre of the disc, although some measurements have been made off-centre[23]. In cadaveric discs it is possible either to use several parallel profiles or expand two pairs of perpendicular profiles[11] to, say, profiles at every 15°. One must be careful, however, not to perturb the disc either by prolonged loading or damage through repeated puncture of the annulus. Should this type of measurement be made it will be possible to map out the overall internal loading of the disc. This will enable the total load acting on the disc to be calculated, after subtraction of the pre-loading which results from the swelling of the proteoglycan matrix. This will allow the relative loading of the disc and facet joints to be determined without resort to crude remove and repeat type experiments. At present such experiments are the only way that the relative loading can be determined, but naturally the act of removal of the facet joints will affect the mechanical of the whole segment and thus introduce some artefact into the measurement.

Most disc profilometry has been performed on cadaveric discs. This has improved our understanding of these structures and how they behave under laboratory loading. The clinical relevance such loading has been determined by a relatively small number of measurements of disc pressure *in-vivo*[24-26]. If stress profiles were measured *in-vivo*, they would provide even more information concerning the internal mechanics of intervertebral discs. A problem of *in-vivo* measurement is that the spine and therefore the discs are continually loaded by the back muscles. This loading is not constant with time, and since profile measurements take a finite time to complete it is possible that temporal changes in load will be confused with spatial variations leading to artefact. Because of this danger it has only been possible to measure stress profiles *in-vivo* in relaxed supine subjects[27].

In conclusion, the use of stress profilometry has already increased our understanding of the internal mechanics underlying the normal and abnormal function of intervertebral discs. It has proved to be a useful tool to monitor the effects of damage and surgical intervention. There are still many aspects of intervertebral disc mechanics which can be illuminated by the further development of stress profilometry.

5. References

1.	A. Naylor and D.L. Snare, *Prelim. Report Brit. Med. J.* **2** (1951) 975.
2.	A.L. Nachemson, *Acta. Orthop. Scand.* **Supp 43** (1960) 1-104.
3.	M. Panjabi, M. Brown, S. Lindahl, L. Irstam and M. Hermens, *Spine* **13** (1988) 913-917.
4.	K. Takashi, S. Inoue, S. Takada, H. Nishiyama, M. Mimura and Y. Wada, *Spine* **11** (1986) 617-620.
5.	W.F. Merriam, R.C. Quinnell, H.R. Stockdale and D.S. Willis, *Spine* **9** (1984) 405-408.
6.	H. Okushima, *Arch. Jpn. Chir.* **39** (1970) 45-57.
7.	A.A. El-Bohy, King-H. Yang and A.I. King, *J. Biomech.* **22** (1989) 931-941.
8.	D.S. McNally, M.A. Adams and A.E. Goodship, *J. Biomed. Eng.* **14** (1992) 495-498.
9.	D.J. Griffiths, *Urodynamics: The mechanics and hydrodynamics of the lower urinary tract* (Adam Hilger Ltd, Bristol, 1980) pp. 66-75.
10.	D. Griffiths, *Phys. Med. Biol.* **30** (1985) 951-963.
11.	D.S. McNally and M.A. Adams, *Spine* **17** (1992) 66-73.
12.	D.S. McNally and R.G.C. Arridge, *J. Biomech.* **28** (1994) .
13.	M.A. Adams, D.S. McNally, H. Chinn and P. Dolan, *Clin. Biomech.* **9** (1994) 5-14.
14.	A.L. Nachemson, *Acta. Orthop. Scand.* **33** (1963) 183-207.
15.	M.A. Adams and P. Dolan, *J. Biomech.* **24** (1991) 117-126.
16.	P. Brinckmann and H. Grootenboer, *Spine* **16** (1991) 641-646.
17.	M.A. Adams, D.S. McNally and A.E. Goodship, *Euro. Spine J.* **1** (1993) 214-221.
18.	R.B. Dunlop, M.A. Adams and W.C. Hutton, *J. Bone Joint Surg.* **66-B** (1984) 706-710.
19.	M.A. Adams and W.C. Hutton, *Spine* **7** (1982) 184-191.
20.	S.J. Gordon, King-H. Yang, P.J. Mayer, A.H. Mace, V.L. Kish and E.L. Radin, *Spine* **16** (1991) 450-456.
21.	D.S. McNally, M.A. Adams and A.E. Goodship, *Spine* **18** (1993) 1525-1530.
22.	D.W.L. Hukins, *Proc. R. Soc. Lond.* **249** (1992) 281-285.
23.	N.R. Ordway, Z.H. Han, Q.B. Bao, M. Itoh, B.M. Pascussi, H.A. Yuan and W.T. Edwards, *Trans. Orthop. Res. Soc.* **19** (1994) 136.
24.	A.L. Nachemson and G. Elfstrom, *Scand. J. Rehabil. Med.* **Supp 1** (1970) 1-40.
25.	A.L. Nachemson and J.M. Morris, *J. Bone Joint Surg.* **46A** (1964) 1077-1092.
26.	A.L. Nachemson, *Acta. Orthop. Scand.* **36** (1965) 418-434.
27.	D.S. McNally, I. Shackleford, R.C. Mulholland and A.E. Goodship, *Trans. Orthop. Res. Soc.* **19** (1994) 735.

CHAPTER 6

THE EXTRACELLULAR MATRIX OF THE INTERVERTEBRAL
DISC: PROTEOGLYCAN BIOCHEMISTRY

B. Johnstone and M.T. Bayliss

1. Introduction

The functional properties of intervertebral disc tissues depend largely upon the structure of their extracellular matrices. Therefore, knowledge of the content, organization and interactions of the molecules within these matrices is vital for the characterization of disc pathologies and for the determination of their aetiology. Apart from water, the major extracellular components of all disc tissues are proteoglycans, collagens and the non-collagenous proteins. In this chapter we will concentrate on recent advances in our knowledge of the biochemistry of proteoglycans. For more general reviews of disc biochemistry the reader should consult recent publications[1,2].

2. Proteoglycans - general description

Proteoglycans are a family of glycoproteins found intracellularly, associated with the cell surface and in the extracellular matrix of all tissues studied[3,4]. They are very diverse in structure and function and are grouped together because of the type of glycosylation they possess; they consist of a protein core to which is attached at least one glycosaminoglycan chain. Glycosaminoglycan chains consist of repeating disaccharides, which vary in their constituent monosaccharides, sulphation patterns and chain lengths. The core proteins are equally diverse. In this chapter we shall discuss our studies on the extracellular matrix (interstitial) proteoglycans of intervertebral disc tissues. This group can be divided into so-called 'large' and 'small' proteoglycans[5].

3. Large interstitial proteoglycans of the intervertebral disc

3.1. General structure

The large aggregating proteoglycans are the major type found in all the disc tissues (annulus, nucleus and end plate). These were originally considered to be similar to aggrecan, the major aggregating proteoglycan of articular cartilage, although important differences have been described (see below). It is now known that aggrecan is a member of a sub-family of large aggregating proteoglycans, but exactly which types exist in the disc is still unknown.

Aggrecan is so named because of its ability to form large aggregates with hyaluronan chains, another glycosaminoglycan which is not associated with a core protein[6]. Aggrecan consists of a protein core of over 200,000 molecular weight to which chondroitin sulphate and keratan sulphate chains and N- and O-linked oligosaccharides are covalently attached. The protein core contains three globular domains (termed G1, G2 and G3) and it is the G1 domain that is involved in the binding of hyaluronan. The major portion of the molecule lies between the G2 and G3 domains and consists of two regions substituted with chondroitin sulphate and keratan sulphate chains. The chondroitin sulphate chains are associated with the large extended region of the molecule which contains over half of the amino acids. Keratan sulphate chains are also attached in this region of the molecule and in the G1-G2 globular region, but the highest concentration of keratan sulphate is in the region of the molecule between the G2 domain and the chondroitin sulphate-rich.

Several studies have shown that the large proteoglycan of the disc resembles aggrecan, the large proteoglycan of articular cartilage[1,2]. They have similar chondroitin sulphate-rich and keratan sulphate-rich domains and also possess the specific N-terminal globular region of the protein core (G1) which enables them to form large aggregates with hyaluronan and link protein. However, tissue specific differences have been observed in the composition, molecular dimensions and the functional properties (aggregation) of disc proteoglycans which depend on the topographical location (annulus vs.nucleus) and the age of the specimen. For example, the concentration of keratan sulphate in the nucleus is always greater than that of the annulus; in fact, the concentration of keratan sulphate in the adult nucleus pulposus is the highest found in any connective tissue[7,8,9]. However, the proportion of keratan sulphate relative to chondroitin sulphate increases with age in both cartilage and the intervertebral disc, but at all ages studied it is higher in the disc[2]. In addition, the mean length of the disc keratan sulphate chain is 2-3 times greater than that of articular cartilage, but the functional significance of keratan sulphate is not known. Heinegård has noted that the keratan sulphate-rich region forms a rigid, extended structure that creates a space between the hyaluronan and the chondroitin sulphate-rich region[10], and that this space has dimensions similar to the diameter of the collagen fibres. It has been suggested that an aggregate might form a 'structural pore' for other matrix molecules to pass through. However, whilst this may be feasible for the keratan sulphate-rich region of cartilage, the same structural arrangement may not apply in the disc since the keratan sulphate chains are as long as the chondroitin sulphate chains which would leave no 'open-pore'.

3.2. Ageing and biosynthesis

As articular cartilage ages there is an increase in the proportion of large proteoglycans that cannot aggregate. This is also apparent in the disc and the proportion is always greater than in articular cartilage at any age and increases to much higher levels than is ever seen in cartilage (Figure 1).

Although aggrecan exhibits marked polydispersity in molecular weight and composition, structurally distinct proteoglycan sub-populations have been identified in cartilage from a number of species[11]. In the adult human intervertebral disc, there are also at least two aggregating and three non-aggregating large proteoglycan populations, which differ in electrophoretic mobility and hydrodynamic size[12,13]. It is generally accepted that many of the changes in aggrecan structure are a consequence of enzymatic cleavage in the extracellular matrix and thus, the high content of non-aggregating, large

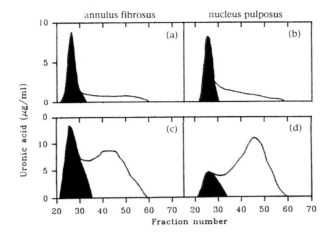

Figure 1. Sepharose CL-2B elution profiles of purified proteoglycans from (a,b) newborn and (c,d) 60 year old annulus fibrosus and nucleus pulposus. The shaded areas represent aggregated proteoglycans.

proteoglycan in the disc represents turnover products that accumulate because of the relatively long pathway for diffusion which exists in the tissue. It is not known, however, what effect changes in the pattern of synthesis may have on proteoglycan composition and structure. *In-vivo* data on proteoglycan synthesis in the disc have been obtained for some animal species[14-17], but only recently has it been possible to measure synthesis in the human disc with any confidence by using a novel *in-vitro* method which controls swelling and proteoglycan loss[18,19]. We have used this technique to investigate the effects of age, topography and pathology on the general synthesis of disc proteoglycans, and on the structure of the newly synthesized, large proteoglycans, comparing them with the proteoglycans pre-existing in the tissue.

Prior to our studies the structure and extracellular assembly of newly-synthesized, human disc proteoglycans had only been investigated once before[20] in a single sample of human nucleus pulposus, and in that study no attempt was made to control tissue structure during culture. Results of our studies on human discs of many ages indicated that there were significant age-related changes in the newly-synthesized large proteoglycans[21]. The majority of newly-synthesized large proteoglycans from newborn discs were extracted in a form capable of aggregation (Figure 2). In young, postnatal discs, however, there was a significant decrease in aggregation and, even though there was considerable variation between specimens, aggregation was reduced to a far greater extent in the extracts of all adult discs. The extracellular mechanism(s) by which aggrecan is consolidated into stable aggregates *in situ* is poorly understood. In adult articular cartilage it has been shown that extracellular maturation of the hyaluronan binding-region (G1) of newly synthesized aggrecan occurs over a relatively long period of time in culture[22,23]. This process, which appears to involve the formation of intra-

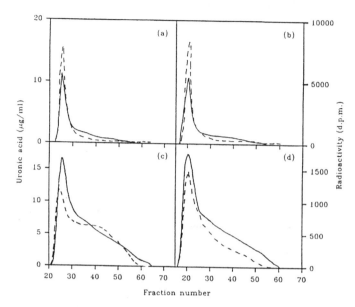

Figure 2. Sepharose CL-2B elution profiles of (-----) newly synthesized and (—) endogenous proteoglycans from slices of newborn (a,b) and 73 year old (c,d) annulus fibrosus which had been pulse-labelled with ³⁵S-sulphate for 4 hours (a,c) and then subjected to non-radioactive chase-culture (b,d) for a further 18 hours.

molecular disulphide bonds in G1[24,25], is essential for the conversion of aggrecan from a molecule with a low-affinity to one with a high-affinity for hyaluronan. It has been postulated that this may be one way of enabling aggrecan to escape the hyaluronan-rich pericellular zone before attaining its full aggregating potential in the intercellular space. Using pulse-chase radiolabelling we showed that this mechanism is also active in adult disc (Figure 2). However, in newborn and immature discs, newly synthesized, large proteoglycans attained full aggregating potential during the initial 4 hour pulse-culture suggesting that either the process of maturation is absent or occurs at a much faster rate. The latter explanation seems the most likely and is consistent with the higher rate of proteoglycan synthesis in discs of this age[26], and also with the need for a more rapid deposition of extracellular matrix during growth and development.

3.3. Structural heterogeneity

Our findings confirmed that a single, high molecular weight, proteoglycan monomer is the major product synthesized at all ages by the cells of the intervertebral disc. The assumption is that this molecule is then converted into the lower molecular weight, faster migrating forms, by proteolytic degradation of the C-terminal chondroitin sulphate-rich region of the protein core, in the extracellular space. Subsequent cleavage of the N-terminal regions during the relatively long time the proteoglycan is resident in the tissue, would then generate the heterogeneous mixture of molecules that have lost their capacity to interact with hyaluronan. Attempts to confirm this hypothesis by performing short-term, pulse-chase experiments were unsuccessful because of the long half-life of the monomer, but this is still the most likely explanation for the decrease in size and increase in concentration of partially degraded, non-aggregating proteoglycans during aging.

Two observations that we have made, however, suggest that this is not necessarily the only explanation and that synthetic processes also contribute to the age changes. Firstly, the aggregating proteoglycan synthesized by newborn disc, has a hydrodynamic size greater than that synthesized by adult disc. Secondly, when adult disc was subdivided into different regions from the outer annulus to the nucleus pulposus it was observed that in some regions more than one ^{35}S-labelled product was synthesized during the initial 4 hour pulse (Figure 3). A subsequent chase-culture of these slices indicated that there was no redistribution of the ^{35}S-labelled bands, confirming that they did not arise from proteolytic degradation during the 4 hour pulse culture. Thus, we now have evidence of a direct contribution of biosynthesis to these structural changes.

Intracellular processes which would result in multiple synthetic products include variable splicing of the mRNA for the proteoglycan core protein. This has been observed for aggrecan synthesised by articular cartilage chondrocytes[27], but it was limited to the C-terminal, G3 region of the protein and therefore is unlikely to play a significant role in producing the extensive changes observed in the molecular size of the extracellular pool. Similarly, variation in glycosylation of the core protein would also change the hydrodynamic size and electrophoretic mobility. Chondroitin sulphate chain size was constant during ageing, but the number of chains on different core proteins may well have varied. Moreover, as discussed earlier there is considerable evidence for age-related changes in the keratan sulphate and chondroitin sulphate content of the endogenous proteoglycan pool, and variation in substitution of the newly synthesized molecules is also possible.

Outer Annulus   Inner Annulus

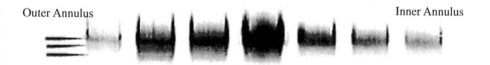

Figure 3. Composite, agarose/polyacrylamide gel electrophoresis of proteoglycans extracted from sagittal slices of radiolabelled annulus fibrosus (45 year old). Individual, newly synthesized aggregating proteoglycan sub-populations were visualised by fluorography (arrows).

3.4. Aggregate stability

Proteoglycan aggregation is accomplished through a non-covalent interaction of the N-terminal globular domain (G1) of core protein with a region of hyaluronan of 10 monosaccharides in length[28,29]. This aggregation is stabilised by link proteins, a 40-50,000 molecular weight glycoprotein (ref. 30 for review). Adult human disc proteoglycan aggregates have been shown to be less stable than those of articular cartilage[31,32]. Furthermore, the link protein of adult discs is much more degraded than that of both young discs and articular cartilage[33,34]. We examined the stability of human disc, large proteoglycan aggregates by adding a large excess of oligosaccharides derived from hyaluronan which dissociate non-link stabilized aggregates by competing with endogenous hyaluronan chains for the binding of aggrecan. Both endogenous and newly-synthesized proteoglycan aggregates purified from foetal annulus were unaffected and remained fully aggregated (Figure 4). Similarly, only a small proportion of aggregate from the 15 month-old disc was dissociated, whereas adult disc proteoglycan aggregates were almost completely dissociated. This age-related decrease in aggregate stability could be due to changes in the quantity and/or quality of disc link protein. Whilst earlier work suggested that there was less abundance of link protein in adult discs, it has been shown more recently that there is no such deficiency[34] and that adult disc link protein is very fragmented.

3.5. General comments

Aggrecan is now known to be one of several members of a proteoglycan sub-family capable of aggregation with hyaluronan[10]. We know that aggrecan is made in the disc ,but we do not know whether other aggregating proteoglycans are also present. Versican, another member of this sub-family, was originally purified and characterized from fibroblast cultures[35]. It contains a N-terminal hyaluronan binding domain homologous to aggrecan G1 and a G3-like domain, however, it has no G2 domain. It is also substituted with chondroitin sulphate, but to a much lesser degree than aggrecan, and does not contain keratan sulphate. Whilst it was initially thought that this proteoglycan represented the fibrous tissue equivalent of aggrecan it appears that this is an over simplification.

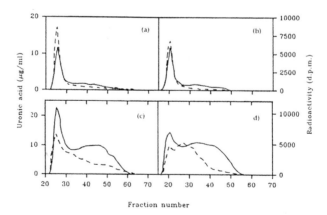

Figure 4. Sepharose Cl-2B elution profiles of (-----) newly synthesized and (—) endogenous proteoglycans from (a,b) 15 month old and (c,d) 55 year old annulus fibrosus treated (a,c) and untreated (b,d) with oligosaccharides of hyaluronan.

For example, although the aortic intima makes versican with the characteristic structure and composition one expects for this molecule, tendon and sclera contain a large proteoglycan with a glycosaminoglycan substitution similar to versican, but lacking the G domain[36]. Since the outer annulus fibrosus is more like fibrocartilage than hyaline cartilage and its cells are much more fibroblast-like, it is possible that other large aggregating proteoglycans of the fibrous tissue-type are present there. In a preliminary report, Johnstone *et al.*[37] found evidence of a versican-like proteoglycan in the outer annulus of human discs. Further work on this proteoglycan is in progress.

4. Small interstitial proteoglycans of the intervertebral disc

4.1. General structure

The core proteins of this proteoglycan sub-family are all members of a larger family of leucine-rich molecules (ref. 38 for recent review). Much of the leucine is contained within amino acid repeats that have the consensus sequence of Leu-X-X-Leu-X-Leu-X-X-Asn-X-Leu-Ser/Thr-X-Leu. The different members of the small proteoglycan sub-family all contain various numbers of this repeating sequence. They can be classified according to the types of glycosaminoglycans attached to the genetically distinct core proteins: biglycan, decorin, proteoglycan-Lb and proteoglycan-100 contain either dermatan sulphate or chondroitin sulphate whereas lumican and fibromodulin contain keratan sulphate

Biglycan and decorin are dermatan/chondroitin sulphate small proteoglycans that have been well-characterized in many connective tissues (ref. 39 for review). These low molecular weight proteoglycans account for only a small proportion of the total mass of proteoglycans present in cartilaginous tissues, however, they may be present in similar molar proportions to the large aggregating proteoglycans[40]. Despite high structural homology it appears that biglycan and decorin have different functions. For example, in tendon, skin, sclera and cornea,decorin has been shown to be specifically associated with the d-band of collagen fibrils[41], and the decorin from tendon can inhibit the rate of type I and type II collagen fibrillogenesis *in vitro*[42,43], whereas biglycan has no effect. Bianco *et al.*[44] have detected decorin mRNA in the annulus and nucleus of a 14-17 week-old human foetus using *in situ* hybridization. The expressed protein was also immunolocalized. In contrast, no message or immunolocalization of biglycan was observed in this study. The exact function(s) of biglycan are unknown, but it is interesting to note that like fibromodulin and decorin, it can bind TGF-β, suggesting a significant role for these molecules in tissue repair[45].

4.2. Tissue distribution and structural heterogeneity

In studies of human intervertebral discs, Johnstone *et al.*[46] identified decorin and biglycan in annulus fibrosus and end-plate, and to a lesser extent in the nucleus pulposus (Figure 5). Immunochemical analyses with an antibody to chondroitin/dermatan sulphate isomers indicated differences in the glycosaminoglycans substituted on glycanated forms of the small proteoglycans found in different disc tissues. Dermatan sulphate was the predominant glycosaminoglycan present on biglycan and decorin in annulus fibrosus extracts whilst chondroitin sulphate was present in both of these proteoglycans isolated

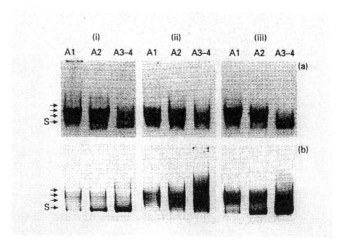

Figure 5. Composite, agarose/polyacrylamide gel electrophoresis of CsCl density gradient fractions from a 4 year old disc tissue extract. Gradient fractions A1, A2 and A3 of decreasing density, from (i) annulus, (ii) nucleus and (iii) end-plate were fractionated on the gels and proteoglycan were stained (a) with toluidine blue and immunolocalised (b) with monoclonal antibody 2-B-6 after Western blotting. The three unlabelled arrows mark the large proteoglycans and the arrow labelled S marks the small proteoglycans biglycan and decorin.

from cartilage end-plate. This finding raises an important structural difference between the cartilage end-plate of the disc and articular cartilage. The composition of the extracellular matrix of the intervertebral disc, cartilage end-plate, has been assumed tobe like that of articular cartilage[47,48]. However, morphological studies have reported structural differences between the two tissues, *e.g.* the collagen fibres of the end-plate join the annulus fibrosus and it is obvious that the arrangement of cells is very different from that of articular cartilage, in that no change in cell size,shape or columnar arrangement is evident towards the bone in the mature end-plate[49]. Furthermore, biochemical studies indicate that both the large proteoglycans[50,51] and the collagens[52] are different to those from articular cartilage. Dermatan sulphate-containing, small proteoglycans are the prevalent form of decorin and biglycan found in articular cartilage[53]. It appears that those of the cartilage end-plate contain only chondroitin sulphate. Collectively, these data emphasize that the cartilage end-plate should be considered a connective tissue which is biochemically and morphologically distinct from articular cartilage.

In addition to the glycosaminoglycan (or glycanated) forms of biglycan and decorin, Johnstone *et al.*[46] also found two non-glycanated forms of both biglycan and decorin in all three regions of the intervertebral disc. The concentration of these components increased with age and their presence is consistent with the hypothesis that some of the non-glycanated forms of decorin and biglycan are degradation products of native precursors. Non-glycanated forms of decorin have been detected in extracts of human and porcine articular cartilage[54,55] and adult human skin[56]. Koob and Horoschak[57] also found a non-glycanated form of decorin in several bovine connective tissues and suggested that this was a degradation product of the glycanated form. They also reported a second minor immunoreactive non-glycanated form but did not characterize it further. Both glycanated and non-glycanated forms of decorin were extractable under the same conditions, indicating that they were both associated with collagen fibrils, a plausible finding since the glycosaminoglycan chain is not required for collagen binding[43,58-60]. There may be functional differences related to the distinct glycosylation patterns of the decorin from different tissues. If this is so, then the removal of the glycosaminoglycan chain-bearing portion of decorin may alter its function in organizing collagen and thereby alter the physiological function of the tissue. The low concentration of glycanated or non-glycanated decorin in the nucleus pulposus supports this hypothesis, since the nucleus contains a random array of collagen fibrils. However, since the nucleus contains much less collagen than the annulus it may also have proportionately less decorin. Thus, the molar ratio of decorin to collagen may be similar to the annulus.

It is still unknown whether or not the two non-glycanated forms of biglycan are degradation products or are synthesized as such. There is some evidence supporting the notion of the synthesis of undersubstituted forms of biglycan: during N-terminal peptide sequencing of biglycan isolated from bovine articular cartilage Neame *et al.*[61] found that approximately 10% of the serine at both of the glycosaminoglycan attachment positions were unsubstituted indicating that biglycan could exist in a form that has only one glycosaminoglycan chain. Furthermore, Jarvelainen *et al.*[62] immunoprecipitated two populations of glycanated biglycan from cultures of bovine aortic and human umbilical vein endothelial cells. One of these had the mobility predicted for biglycan with a single glycosaminoglycan chain. Thus, it is possible that a non-glycanated form of biglycan could also be produced.

Fibromodulin and lumican are two small proteoglycans that contain keratan sulphate (ref. 38 for review). The keratan sulphate is attached to the core protein via an N-glycosidic linkage from N-acetylglucosamine to asparagine residues[63,64]. Like decorin, both proteoglycans have been found to influence collagen fibrillogenesis. Fibromodulin is present in many tissues including cartilage. Lumican, in its proteoglycan form, appears to be exclusive to the cornea. Other forms of lumican have been found in other tissues, but they lack the keratan sulphate substitution of their N-linked oligosaccharides. Immunolocation and immunohistochemical staining of fibromodulin and lumican in porcine intervertebral disc tissues has been reported[65], but more work is required to confirm this preliminary data and lumican has also been found in the human intervertebral disc (B. Johnstone, unpublished results).

5. Conclusions

The anatomical features of the intervertebral disc are a product of the interaction of diverse tissue structures which combine to provide each segment with its unique biomechanical properties. The morphological characteristics of each region of the disc are a reflection of the highly organised, macromolecular components of the extracellular matrix. It is becoming increasingly apparent that in order to appreciate the pathological processes leading to disc disorders, we must increase our knowledge of these components and their interactions as well as improving our understanding of the cells which synthesize and degrade them.

6. References

1.   M.T. Bayliss and B. Johnstone, in *The lumbar spine and back pain*, ed. M.I.V. Jayson (Churchill Livingstone, Edinburgh, 1992).

2.   C.A. McDevitt, in *Biology of the intervertebral disc*, ed. P. Ghosh (CRC Press Inc., Boca Raton. 1988).

3.   T.E. Hardingham and A.J. Fosang, *FASEB J.* **6** (1992) 861.

4.   P.J. Neame, in *Joint cartilage degradation. Basic and clinical aspects*, ed. J.F. Woessner and D.S. Howell (Marcel Dekker, Inc., New York. 1993).

5.   D. Heinegård, A. Bjorne-Persson, L. Cöster, A. Franzèn, S. Gardell, A. Malmström, M. Paulsson, R. Sandfalk and K. Vogel, *Biochem. J.* **230** (1985).

6.   K. Doege, C. Rhodes, M. Sasaki, J.R. Hassell and J. Yamada, in *Extracellular matrix genes*, ed, L. Sandell and C. Boyd (Academic Press, New York. 1990).

7.   C. Antonopoulos, L. Fransson, S. Gardell and D. Heinegård, *Acta. Chem. Scand.* **1** (1969) 23.

8.   R.H. Pearce and B.J. Grimmer, *Biochem. J.* **157** (1973) 753.

9.   M.R. Jahnke and C.A. McDevitt, *Biochem. J.* **251** (1988)347.

10. D. Heinegård and Å. Oldberg, in *Connective tissue and its heritable disorders*, (Wiley-Liss, Inc. 1993).

11. L.C. Rosenberg and J.A. Buckwalter, in *Articular cartilage biochemistry*, ed, K. E. York. (1986).

12. J.L. DiFabio, R.H. Pearce, B. Caterson and C. Hughes, *Biochem. J.* **244** (1987) 27.

13. M.R. Jahnke and C.A. McDevitt, *Biochem .J.* **251** (1988) 347.

14. E.A. Davidson and W. Small, *Biochim. Biophys. Acta.* **69** (1963) 445.

15. L.S. Lohmander, C.A. Antonopoulos and U. Friberg, *Biochim. Biophys. Acta.* **304** (1973) 430.

16. J.P.G. Urban, S. Holm, A. Maroudas, *Biorheology* 15 (1978) 203.

17. G. Venn and R.M. Mason, *Biochem. J.* **215** (1983) 217.

18. M.T. Bayliss, B. Johnstone and J.P. O'Brien, *Spine* 13 (1988) 972.

19. M.T. Bayliss, J.P.G. Urban, B. Johnstone and S. Holm, *J. Orthop. Res.* **4** (1986) 10.

20. T.R. Oegema, D.S. Bradford and K.M. Cooper, *J. Biol. Chem.* **254** (1979) 10579.

21. B. Johnstone and M.T. Bayliss, *Spine* (In press).
22. M.T. Bayliss, G.D. Ridgway and S.Y. Ali, *Biochem. J.* **215** (1983) 705.
23. T.R. Oegema, *Nature* **288** (1980) 583.
24. A.H.K. Plaas and J.D. Sandy, *Biochem. J.* **234** (1986) 221.
25. J.D. Sandy and A.H.K. Plaas, *Arch. Biochem. Biophys.* 271 (1989) 300.
26. M.T. Bayliss, J.P.G. Urban, B. Johnstone and S. Holm, *J. Orthop. Res.* **4** (1986) 10.
27. C.T. Baldwin, A.M. Reginato and D.J. Prockop, *J. Biol. Chem.* **264** (1989) 15747.
28. T.E. Hardingham and H. Muir, *Biochem. J.* **135** (1973) 905.
29. V.C. Hascall and D. Heinegård, *J. Biol. Chem.* 249 (1974) 4242.
30. P.J. Neame and F.P. Barry, *Experientia* **49** (1993) 393.
31. A. Tengblad, R.H. Pearce and B.J. Grimmer, *Biochem. J.* **222** (1984) 85.
32. P.J. Donohue, M.R. Jahnke, J.D. Blaha and B, Caterson, *Biochem. J.* 251 (1988) 739.
33. R.H. Pearce, J.M. Mathieson, S.J. Mort and P.J. Roughley, *J. Orthop. Res.* **7** (1989) 861.
34. J. Liu, R.H. Pearce, J.M. Mathieson, P.J. Roughley and J.S. Mort, *Trans. Orthop. Res. Soc.* **18** (1993) 212.
35. D.R. Zimmermann and E. Ruoslahti, *EMBO J.* **8** (1989) 2975.
36. M. Morgelin, M. Paulsson, A. Malmström and D. Heinegård, *J. Biol. Chem.* **264** (1989) 12080.
37. B. Johnstone, S. Roberts and J. Menage, *Trans. Orthop. Res. Soc.* **19** (1994) 132.
38. H. Kresse, H. Hausser and E. Schonherr, *Experientia* **49** (1993) 403.
39 V. Stanescu, *Arth. Rheum.* **20** (1990) 51.
40. P.R. Roughley and R.J. White, *Biochem. J.* **262** (1989) 823.
41. J.E. Scott, *Biochem. J.* **252** (1988) 313.
42. K. Vogel, M. Paulsson and D. Heinegård, *Biochem. J.* **223** (1984) 587.
43. E. Hedbom and D. Heinegård, *J. Biol. Chem.* **264** (1989) 6898.
44. P. Bianco, L.W. Fisher, M.F. Young, J.D. Termine and P. Gehron Robey, *J. Histochem. Cytochem*, **38** (1990) 1549.
45. A. Hildebrand, M. Romaris, L.M. Rasmussen, D. Heinegård, D.R. Twardzik, W.A. Border and E. Ruoslahti, *Biochem. J.* **302** (1994) 527.
46. B. Johnstone, M. Markopoulos, P. Neame and B. Caterson, *Biochem. J.* **292** (1993) 661.
47. D.R. Eyre, *Int. Rev. Conn. Tis. Res.* **8** (1979) 227.
48. S. Ayad and J.B. Weiss, in *The Lumbar Spine and Back Pain.* ed. M.I.V. Jayson (Churchill-Livingstone, Edinburgh 1987).
49. S. Roberts, J. Menage and J.P.G. Urban, *Spine* **14** (1989) 166.
50. P.B Bishop and R.H. Pearce, *J. Orthop. Res.* **11** (1993) 324.
51. M.R. Jahnke and B. Caterson, *Trans. Orthop. Res. Soc.* **11** (1986) 419.
52. S. Roberts, J. Menage, V. Duance, S. Wotton and S. Ayad, *Spine* **16** (1991) 1030.

53. L.C. Rosenberg, H.U. Choi, L-H, Tang, T.L. Johnson, S. Pal, C. Webber, A. Rein and A.R. Poole, *J. Biol. Chem.* **260** (1985) 6304.

54. L.O. Sampaio, M.T. Bayliss, T.E. Hardingham and H. Muir, *Biochem. J.* **254** (1988) 757.

55. P.J. Roughley, R.J. White, M.C. Magny, J. Liu, R.H. Pearce and J.S. Mort, *Biochem. J.* **295** (1993) 421.

56. R. Fleischmajer, L.W. Fisher, E.D. MacDonald, L. Jacobs, J.S. Perlish and J.D. Termine, *J. Struc. Biol.* **106** (1991) 82.

57. T.J. Koob and S.A. Horoschak, *Trans. Orthop. Res. Soc.* **15** (1990) 38.

58. K.G. Vogel, T.J. Koob, L.W. Fisher, *Biochem. Biophys. Res. Comm.* **148** (1987) 658.

59. N. Uldbjerg and C.C. Danielsen, *Biochem. J.* **251** (1988) 643.

60. D.C. Brown and K.G. Vogel, *Matrix* **91** (1989) 468.

61. P.J. Neame, H.U. Choi, and L.C. Rosenberg, *J. Biol. Chem.* **264** (1989) 8653.

62. H.J. Jarvelainen, M.G. Kinsella, T.N. Wight and L.J. Sandell, *J. Biol. Chem.* **266** (1991) 23274.

63. J.R. Hassell, T.C. Blochberger, J.A. Rada, S. Chakravarti and D. Noona, *Adv. Mol. Cell. Biol.* **6** (1993) 69.

64. P. Antonsson, D. Heinegård, and Å. Oldberg, *J. Biol. Chem.* **266** (1991) 16859.

65. M. Markopoulos, B. Johnstone, P. Neame and B. Caterson, *Trans. Orthop. Res. Soc.* **19** (1994) 133.

CHAPTER 7

THE EFFECT OF MECHANICAL STRESS ON CELLULAR ACTIVITY IN THE INTERVERTEBRAL DISC

J.P.G. Urban and K. Puustjarvi

1. Introduction

The major role of the intervertebral discs is mechanical. The discs link the vertebral bodies and transmit loads through the spinal column; because of their flexibility they allow the spinal column to bend, flex and twist. The discs are a specialised cartilage and consist predominantly of an extracellular matrix, the main constituents being water, fibril-forming collagens and the large aggregating proteoglycan aggrecan; together these form 90-95% of the disc matrix, the remaining fraction consisting of small proteoglycans and glycoproteins, and minor collagens[1,2]. It is the composition and organisation of this extracellular matrix which enable the discs to fulfil their mechanical role. The discs also contain cells; they constitute around 1-5% of tissue volume. Throughout life these cells synthesize and turn over the cartilage macromolecules; they are thus ultimately responsible for maintenance of disc composition.

It is now known that mechanical loads can modify matrix composition in cartilaginous tissues, despite their low cellularity and metabolic activity. In articular cartilage in particular many studies have found that cartilage is thickest and proteoglycan concentration highest in areas of cartilage which are habitually subjected to high loads *in vivo*[3,4]. If loads are removed from a joint, cartilage thins and proteoglycans are lost[5-7]. Reloading the joint leads to limited replacement of proteoglycans. Exercise studies have found that *in vivo* alterations in loading pattern lead to changes in cartilage composition and in cell morphology[8,9]. Abnormal loading, after anterior cruciate ligament section for example, can result in disruption of the matrix and development of osteoarthritis[10].

The cells of cartilages also respond to *in vitro* loading, with the response depending on loading pattern. Static loading of articular cartilage explants invariably produces a decrease in matrix synthesis rates, the decrease being proportional to the applied load (reviewed Gray *et al*[11]). The response to cyclic loading however depends on frequency. The same load amplitude depresses synthesis at low frequencies (.001-.01Hz) but stimulates synthesis at higher frequencies (>0.1Hz)[12]. Load also affects the synthesis of other matrix macromolecules such as fibronectin[13].

Since in many respects disc cells are similar to cartilage cells, it is reasonable to suppose that mechanical stress also plays a role in regulating the activity of disc cells. This chapter will review current information on this topic.

2. *In-vivo* studies

2.1. *Animal studies; changes in disc composition with altered loading pattern*

In animal studies, unphysiological mechanical stress patterns have been shown to induce disc degeneration within a few months. Running on a cylinder treadmill was found to reduce the disc height in rats[14,15]. Forced bipedal gait in mice or rats induced degeneration in the nucleus pulposus. The annulus fibrosus became disordered, especially the posterior annulus fibrosus of the lumbar spine. Protrusions and prolapses of the discs were seen and the endplates were irregular in structure. The histological appearance was similar to that seen in aged animals[16-18]. Intensive passive daily two-hour flexion-extension movement in an arc of 100° was shown to induce disc prolapses and degenerative changes in the endplates of young rats within two months[19]. Repetitive flexion-extension movement of rabbit cervical spine induced structural abnormalities of annulus fibrosus and vertebral osteophytes also within two months[20].

In vivo studies have also shown that reduced loading affects the metabolism and composition of the disc. The wet and dry weights of the lumbar discs of the rats flown in COSMOS were significantly smaller and the collagen-to-proteoglycan ratio was significantly higher in the flight group than in the controls[21]. A different model of reduced loading, i.e. fusion of a canine spinal segment, caused a reduction of oxygen consumption rate within three months of fusion, while the oxygen tension level in the disc increased over the same time period. The discs in the fused segment also lost proteoglycan and water progressively. In the discs adjacent to the fused segments, the findings were the opposite, possibly because of enhanced loading[22]. In another study, fusion was shown to lead to alterations in intervertebral disc proteoglycans. The proteoglycan population present after 12 months was larger, particularly in the annulus fibrosus. Net loss of proteoglycans was seen in the nucleus pulposus. In fused segments the synthesis of new proteoglycan was activated, and the structure of the proteoglycans resembled that of immature tissues[23].

The change in activity level does not have to be extreme to affect the cellular activity of the disc. Experiments on dogs have shown that it is possible to stimulate aerobic metabolism of the disc tissue by moderate exercise and spinal movements within three months[24]. Transport of solutes, such as sulphate and glucose, and incorporation of sulphate, a measure of proteoglycan synthesis, were enhanced in the exercised group as compared to a sedentary control group of dogs. The uptake rates of glucose, oxygen and glycogen increased while the production of lactate in the outer annulus fell.

More strenuous exercise however, can have deleterious effects on the disc. In some recent studies on dogs performed in Finland, a strenuous running exercise program was conducted; beagle dogs ran for a year on a treadmill for five days a week. The daily running distance was increased progressively up to 40 km/day, which distance the dogs ran for the last 15 weeks. Examination of the discs showed a decrease in the concentrations of proteoglycans, enhancement of the proteoglycan synthesis rate and a higher level of small proteoglycan-species in the upper thoracic discs; these changes resemble the alterations seen in degeneration of the disc. Similar changes were observed in the cervical discs. However the lumbar and lower thoracic discs were not significantly affected, their proteoglycan properties being similar to those of the sedentary control dogs[25-26]. The activity of enzymes involved in collagen synthesis increased in the thoracic and lumbar posterior annulus fibrosus, and in the lumbar nucleus pulposus of these running dogs[27], though collagen content was unchanged. Running however did not appear to affect collagen crosslinking; no difference was found in the concentration of mature hydroxypyridinium crosslinks of collagen between the two groups.

2.2. Clinical studies on the effect of load on human disc composition and metabolism

There is also some evidence that loading patterns affect human discs. The most convincing evidence comes from the study of scoliosis where there is long-term, altered loading on the intervertebral discs *in vivo*. The composition of the discs has been found to alter; a shift in the ratio of type II/type I collagen in the annulus, an increase in the degree of calcification in the end-plate, and a loss of proteoglycan on the compressed side of the disc have all been reported[21,28-30]. In non-idiopathic scoliosis arising because of cerebral-palsy say, where it is clear that no connective tissue defect exists, the changes in composition and structure are secondary and are induced by altered force pattern across the disc. Although similar changes in disc composition are found in idiopathic scoliosis and it is likely that these too are induced by altered mechanical forces, some defect of connective tissue metabolism in these patients cannot been ruled out.

Levels of activity have been reported to influence on the incidence of back-pain, and thus possibly disc metabolism. For instance, some clinical and epidemiological studies show that physical activity and fitness have a protective effect against back injuries and pain [31,32]. On the other hand, intensive sports activities in adolescence and heavy work are both associated with an increased incidence of low back pain and disc degeneration [33-39].

Prolonged changes in the prevailing levels of mechanical stress on the spine, following from the initiation of an exercise programme, or after a period of inactivity, will affect the spinal musculature. An MRI study found that atrophy of spinal muscles, was more common in adolescents with a low level of leisure-time activity for instance[40]. The muscles of the beagles, running 40 km/day where found to alter; there was a significant transformation of type I to type II muscle fibres in the lumbar spine, and the opposite finding in the thoracic and cervical spine and in the extensors of the elbow joints[41]. Changes in proteoglycan content in the discs, correlated well with changes in muscle fibre type; proteoglycan content increases with an increase in typeII/I ratio and vice versa[41]. This is in agreement with a study which shows an association between the atrophy of type II fibres and disc degeneration in humans[42,43]. Spinal muscle activity and contraction forces have been shown to correlate well with intradiscal pressure[44], thus the same activity carried out by people of differing levels of fitness, will impose different forces on the disc.

2.3. Why in-vitro studies are necessary

The studies outlined above, have shown that mechanical factors can lead to alterations in disc composition and cellular metabolism. However from such *in-vivo* studies, it is very difficult to elucidate the mechanism, or even to see if disc cells, like other cartilage cells, can respond directly to mechanical stress. The level of load on the disc is not known except in general terms. Some forms of exercise, may increase the density of the capillary bed that feeds the disc and thus improve disc nutrition; alternatively exposure to vibration may reduce the peripheral circulation and have the opposite effect. Exercise may also alter the concentration of blood solutes such as glucose and lactic acid. The hormonal status of exercised animals may be different to those of sedentary controls. The concentration of growth factors and cytokines in the blood may also be affected by exercise. The changes seen in the discs thus may arise because the chondrocytes are responding to changes in concentrations of circulating factors, rather than to changes in mechanical stress as such. More precise information on factors which may influence cellular behaviour can really only be obtained from *in vitro* studies.

3. *In-vitro* studies

3.1. *Problems arising when incubating the disc in vitro*

Compared to articular cartilage there have been extraordinarily few studies of disc metabolism *in vitro*; a recent literature search found 7 papers on disc metabolism over the previous 2 decades, compared to over 25 papers on articular cartilage in 1991 alone, using the same search terms[45]. There are several reasons why so few experimental studies have been performed on the disc. For one thing, suitable human disc material is not readily available, while suitable animal discs are expensive. Recently, H. Tsuji and colleagues initiated the use of coccygeal discs[45]. Characterisation of these discs have found that they have similar properties to lumbar spinal discs in terms of their composition, physicochemical behaviour and synthetic activity, and are under considerable compressive load. Much of the recent work on the effects of load on disc metabolism has been carried out on coccygeal discs.

Another problem arises because the disc is difficult to incubate successfully *in vitro* because of swelling and leaching. The disc *in vivo* is always under load from muscle and ligament tensions and from body weight. If the disc is incubated *in vitro* by placing a whole disc or a slice of disc in solution, the osmotic balance of the tissue is disturbed, the disc swells and proteoglycans, and probably other matrix components, leach out, thus changing the environment of the chondrocyte[46-47]; such changes have been shown to have a strong effect on cellular activity. Thus in order to measure metabolic activity in the disc satisfactorily, swelling and leaching need to be prevented. This can be achieved *in vitro* by enclosing the disc explant in a semi-permeable membrane to prevent proteoglycan loss, and by increasing the osmotic pressure of the medium using PEG (polyethylene glycol 20000), an inert high molecular weight solute, to balance the osmotic pressure of the disc proteoglycans and prevent swelling[47]. While this method has proved valuable for short term studies of matrix synthesis *in vitro*[48-49], and has given information on synthesis of proteoglycans in different regions of human disc, it is difficult to use for direct studies on the effect of mechanical load on metabolism because of the viscosity of the PEG medium and because the tissue has to be enclosed in a dialysis sac.

An alternative system for incubating the disc *in vitro* has been developed. Here *in vivo* hydrations are maintained by applying a mechanical stress instead of an osmotic stress to replace the load experienced by the disc *in vivo*; concentrations of metabolites can be kept constant by steady state perfusion to the surface of the disc[50]. This system has been used to study the effect of mechanical loads on disc metabolism.

3.2. *Direct effects of load on cellular activity*

Recent work on disc explants has shown that the cells of the disc can respond directly to applied mechanical load, and that as in other cartilage, the response varies with the applied loading pattern.

3.3. The effect of static load on disc metabolism

When intact bovine coccygeal discs were incubated in a perfusion cell, it was found that cellular activity was varied with the applied load. Protein and proteoglycan synthesis rates were lowest when the load was 0.5 kg. They increased 2-3 fold as the load was raised to 5 to 10 kg, and then fell again as it was further raised to 15 kg. The effect of load on the disc is different to that of other cartilages; in articular, epiphyseal or nasal cartilage, metabolic rates fall monotonically with increase in the level of static load[50].

It has been suggested that the influence of static load on cartilage cells is mediated mainly through the effect of load on tissue hydration[51]. It is thus of interest to observe that in the disc, if hydration is changed osmotically with PEG rather than by increasing mechanical stress, a similar bell-shaped curve was observed[47]. The effect of an increase in static load on the metabolism of the disc under physiological conditions thus appears to depend mainly on the effect of load on disc fluid content.

3.4. The effects of vibration on disc cell metabolism

The effects of vibration on disc metabolism was investigated in pig coccygeal discs[52]. A disc-endplate unit was exposed to sinusoidal vibratory load of 3N superimposed on a static load of 5N for several hours, at frequencies rising to 35 Hz; the resonant frequency of the disc-endplate complex being 11 Hz. Metabolic activity of the different disc regions was measured immediately after exposure to vibration, using the PEG incubation method. Synthesis rates in the annulus seemed relatively unaffected even after exposure to frequencies of 35 Hz; in the nucleus however, synthesis rates were similar to control rates at 3.5Hz, but fell significantly at higher frequencies.

3.5. The effect of hydrostatic pressure on disc cell metabolism

When the disc is loaded in compression, it deforms and bulges radially setting the outer annulus into tension and causing a rise in hydrostatic pressure in the nucleus and inner annulus[33,34]; the extent of the pressure rise depends on the compressive load applied by body weight, muscle activity and ligament tensions[53,54]. Disc metabolism has been shown to be significantly affected by the application of hydrostatic pressure. When disc explants were exposed to physiological levels of pressure (5-25 atmospheres, 0.5-2.5 MPa) for only 20 seconds, synthesis of proteoglycans and proteins was stimulated in the nucleus pulposus, and particularly the inner annulus of human and bovine discs for at least the following 2 hours. Higher pressures (50-100 atmospheres) appeared to inhibit incorporation in these regions. The outer annulus in contrast to the other regions of the disc showed virtually no response to pressure over the range tested (0.5-10 MPa)[55].

4. How does load affect disc metabolism

It is now clear from the evidence discussed briefly above, that altered levels of mechanical stress can affect the activity of disc cells, and thus the composition of the intervertebral disc. There are many possible modulating mechanisms. As discussed briefly above, the effect of changes in level of activity on disc cell metabolism and composition seen *in vivo*, could arise through cellular responses to changes in levels of circulating factors. Indeed there is experimental evidence to show that disc cells respond to changes in growth factor concentrations, to cytokines, and to extracellular lactate[56-58]. The *in vitro* experiments discussed above have now also shown that the cells also respond directly to changes in mechanical stress.

4.1. Effects of changes in hydration and pressure on cells

Studies on the *in vitro* response of articular cartilage to load have indicated that cartilage cells respond not to load as such, but to the load-induced changes in deformation, hydrostatic pressure, fluid and ion content and fluid flow which occur in their immediate environment[59]. Since the response of disc cells appears to be similar to that of cartilage, it seems that the disc cells also respond in a similar manner.

An increase in static loading, above the *in vivo* resting levels leads to a dose dependent fall in synthesis rates in both cartilage and disc. Under this loading regime, fluid is expressed from the tissue and changes in synthesis rates have been related directly to loss of fluid[60]. Fluid loss causes a proportional increase in proteoglycan concentration, leading to an increase in extracellular cation concentrations and osmolality and a decrease in extracellular pH. Low loads will cause the disc, but not cartilage to swell[46], thus also altering the extracellular ionic environment. It now seems that the cells respond to the changes in extracellular ion concentrations, rather than directly to hydration, at least in part[61-63].

Physiological levels of hydrostatic pressure have been found to affect a wide variety of cellular functions, which can frequently be explained by changes in the conformation of membrane-bound or intracellular proteins; cytoskeletal elements in particular are known to be sensitive to hydrostatic pressure[64]. Recent studies have shown that high pressures (> 150 atmospheres) disrupt cytoskeletal elements in chondrocytes[65] which could explain the fall in incorporation at these pressures. The outer annulus of the disc did not appear to respond to physiological levels of hydrostatic pressure. When the disc is loaded, no pressure rise is seen in this region[33], thus previous routine exposures to pressure, as well as cell type, may also determine the pressure response.

4.2. Effect of nutrient levels on disc cell metabolism

While it is clear from the evidence above, that mechanical stress can alter disc cell metabolism directly, mechanical stress can also alter nutrient levels in the disc by affecting the blood supply to the vertebral bodies and annulus periphery. Cellular activity can be modified significantly if supplies of nutrients are altered, by this or other means. The energy supply of the disc is obtained mainly through anaerobic glycolysis; the disc thus produces large amounts of lactate[66]. However the disc does use oxygen. If the oxygen supplied to the disc is reduced for example, oxygen levels fall, particularly in the disc centre[67]. Since the disc exhibits a Pasteur effect, *i.e.* an increase in glycolysis rate at low oxygen concentration, the amount of lactate produced by the disc cells will increase[67]. Both a fall in oxygen levels, and an increase in lactate concentration (*i.e.* a fall in pH) lead to a decrease in the synthesis of proteoglycans and protein[58,68].

It is often stated that the supply of nutrients is increased by 'pumping' fluid in and out of the disc in response the pressure gradients induced by load. Experimental and theoretical work has shown that for small molecules such as the major nutrients and metabolic substrates such as glucose, oxyen, sulphate and amino-acids, this effect is negligble. For instance *in vivo* transport of sulphate into the disc of dogs was the same whether the animals were anaesthetized (relaxed, fluid moving into the disc) or if they were running (discs loaded, fluid moving out of the disc)[69]. Transport of these nutrients thus occurs mainly by diffusion. Indeed, if nutrients depended on fluid flow for transport into the disc, the tissue would be deprived of oxygen and glucose for example, during the time fluid was flowing from rather than into the disc - *i.e.* during the periods of activity, or for around 16 out of 24 hours. Transport of large molecules, such as growth factors or cytokines may however be affected by 'pumping'[70].

5. Conclusions

Changes in the prevailing levels of applied mechanical load undoubtedly affect cellular activity and hence lead to changes in disc composition and thus to its mechanical behaviour. However the signals reaching the disc as a consequence of load application are very complicated. Prolonged changes in the level of activity can alter spinal musculature and thus affect the actual levels of intradiscal pressure. As in other cartilaginous tissues, the disc cells respond to changes in pressure and to the loss of fluid in their environment arising from load application. Load may also alter nutrient supply by affecting circulation around the disc. In addition, exercise may change concentrations of factors such as hormones or lactate which can also modify disc cell activity. The relative importance of these different signals, and interactions between them still remain to be elucidated.

6. Acknowledgements

We thank the Arthritis and Rheumatism Council (U0501) and the Finnish Medical Academy for support.

7. References

1. D.R. Eyre, B. Caterson, P. Benya *et al.*, in: *New Perspectives on Low Back Pain*, ed. S. Gordon and J. Frymoyer, (Am. Inst. Orthop. Surg., Philadeplhia (1991).
2. T.R Oegema, *Clinics in Sports Medicine* **12** (1993) 419.
3. S. Roberts, B. Weightman, J.P.G. Urban, and D. Chapell, *J. Bone Joint Surg.* **68-B** (1986) 278.
4. S.D Slowman and K.D. Brandt, *Arthr. Rheum.* **29** (1986) 88.
5. M. Palmoski, R.A. Colyer and K.D. Brandt, *Arthr. Rheum.* **23** (1980) 325.
6. M. Palmoski, E. Perricone and K.D. Brandt, *Arthr. Rheum.* **22** (1979) 508.
7. J. Jurvelin, H. Helminen, S. Lauritsalo *et al.*, *Acta Anat.* **122** (1985) 62.

8.   K. Paukkonen, K. Selkainaho, J. Jurvelin and H.J. Helminen, *J. Anat.* **142** (1985) 13.

9.   I. Kiviranta, M. Tammi, J. Jurvelin, J. Arokoski, A-M. Säämanen and H. Helminen, *J. Orthop. Res.* **6** (1988) 188.

10.   H. Muir and S.L. Carney, in *Joint Loading: biology and health of articular structures*, ed. H.J. Helminen, I. Kiviranta, M.Tammi, A-M. Säämanen, K. Paukkonen and J. Jurvelin, (J. Wright, Bristol, 1988) p.47.

11.   M. Gray, A. Pizzanelli, A. Grodzinsky and R. Lee, *J. Orthop. Res.* **6** (1988) 777.

12.   R.L-Y. Sah, Y-J. Kim, J-Y.H. Doong, A. Plaas and J. Sandy, *J. Orthop. Res.* **7** (1989) 619.

13.   N. Burton-Wurster, M. Vernier-Singer, T. Farquhar and G. Lust, *J. Orthop. Res.* **11** (1993) 717.

14.   I. Ziv and H.J. Neufeld, *Trans. Orthop. Res. Soc.* **18** (1993) 209.

15.   H.J. Neufeld, *Spine* **17** (1992) 811.

16.   K. Yamada, *J. Exp. Med.* **8** (1962) 350.

17.   J. Cassidy, M. Yong-Hing, W. Kirkaldy-Willis and A. Wilkinson, *Spine* **13** (1988) 301.

18.   M. Higuchi, K. Abe and K. Kaneda, *Clin. Orthop.* **175** (1983) 251.

19.   M. Revel, C. Andre-Deshays, B. Roudier, G. Hamard and B. Amor, *Clin. Orthop.* **279** (1992) 303.

20.   E. Wada, S. Ebara, S. Susumu and K. Ono, *Spine* **17** (1992) S1.

21.   A. Pedrini-Mille, J.A. Maynard, G.N. Durnova, A.S. Kaplansky, V.A. Pedrini and C.B. Chung, *J. Appl. Physiol.* **73 (suppl)** (1992) S26.

22.   S. Holm, and A. Nachemson, *Clin. Orthop.* **169** (1982) 243.

23.   T-K. Cole, D. Burkhardt, P. Ghosh, M. Ryan and T.K.F. Taylor, *J. Orthop. Res.* **3** (1985) 277.

24.   S. Holm and A. Nachemson, *Spine* **8** (1983) 866.

25.   K. Puustjarvi, M. Lammi, I. Kiviranta, H.J. Helminen and M. Tammi, *J. Orthop. Res.* **11** (1993) 738.

26.   K. Puustjarvi, T. Takala, W. Wang, M. Tammi, H.J. Helminen and R. Inkinen, *Connect. Tiss. Res.* **30** (1993) 1.

27.   K. Puustjarvi, T. Takala, W. Wang, M. Tammi, H.J. Helminen and Kovanen, *Eur. Spine. J.* **2** (1993) 126.

28.   J. Melrose, K.R. Gurr, T-C. Cole, A. Darvodelsky, P. Ghosh and T.K.F. Taylor, *J. Orthop. Res.* **9** (1991) 68.

29.   D. Brickley-Parsons and M. Glimcher, *Spine* **9** (1984) 148.

30.   H.K. Beard, R. Ryvar, R. Brown and H. Muir, *Immunology* **41** (1980) 491.

31.   W. Cats-Baril and J. W. Frymoyer, *Spine* **16** (1991) 605.

32.   R.A. Deyo and J.E. Bass, *Spine* **14** (1989) 501.

33.   D.S. McNally and M.A. Adams, *Spine* **17** (1992) 66.

34.   A. Nachemson, *Acta Orthop. Scand.* **suppl 43** (1960) 1.

35.   F. Balaque, G. Dutoit and M. Waldburger, *Scand. J. Rehabil. Med.* **20** (1988) 175.

36.   J.J. Salminen, P. Maki, A. Oksanenm and Penti, J. *Spine* **17** (1992) 405.

37. L. Sward, M. Hellstrom, B. Jacobsson and L. Peterson, *Spine* **15** (1990) 124.
38. M. Hellstrom, B. Jakobsson, L. Sward and Peterson, L. *Act. Radiol.* **31** (1994) 127.
39. H. Riihimaki, *Back disorders in relation to heavy physical work*, University of Helsinki, 1990.
40. J.J. Salminen, M.O. Erkintalo-Terti and H.E.K. Paajanen, *J. Spinal Disorders* **6** (1993) 386.
41. K. Puustjarvi, H.J. Helminen and M. Tammi, *Trans. Orthop. Res. Soc.* **19** (1994)
42. M.W. Fidler, R.L. Jowett and J.D.G. Troup, *J. Bone Joint Surg.* **57B** (1975) 220.
43. M. Mattila, M. Hurme, H. Alaranta *et al*,. *Spine* **11** (1986) 732.
44. A. Schultz, G.B.J. Andersson, R. Ortengren, K. Haderspeck and A. Nachemson, *J. Bone Joint Surg.* **64A** (1982) 713.
45. H. Ohshima, H. Ishihara, H. Tsuji, and J.P.G. Urban, *J. Orthop. Res.* (1993) **11** 332.
46. J.P.G. Urban and A. Maroudas, *Connect. Tiss. Res.* **9** (1981) 1.
47. M.T. Bayliss, J.P.G. Urban, B. Johnstone and S. Holm, *J. Orthop. Res.* **4** (1986) 10.
48. M.T. Bayliss, B. Johnstone and J.P. O'Brien, *Spine* **13** (1988) 972.
49. B. Johnstone and M.T. Bayliss, *Spine* **in press** (1994)
50. H. Ohshima, J.P.G. Urban and D.H. Bergel, *J. Orthop. Res.* **in press** (1994)
51. J.P.G. Urban and A.S. Hall, In: *The Mechanics of Swelling. From Clays to Living Cells and Tissues*, ed. T.K.Karalis. (Springer, 1992) 513.
52. H. Ishihara, H. Tsuji, H. Ohshima and N. Terahata, *Spine* **17(suppl)** (1992) 7.
53. A. Nachemson and G. Elfstrom, *Scand. J. Rehabil. Med.* **2 (suppl 1)** (1970) 1.
54. A. Nachemson, in *The Lumbar Spine and Back Pain*, ed. M.I.V. Jayson, (Churchill Livingstone, Edinburgh 1987), p.191.
55. H. Ishihara, J.P.G. Urban and A.S. Hall, *J. Physiol.* **467** P214
56. J.P. Thompson, T.R. Oegema and D.S. Bradford, *Spine* **16** (1991) 253.
57. J. Liu, P.J. Roughley and J.S. Mort, *J. Orthop. Res.* **9** (1991) 568.
58. H. Ohshima and J.P.G. Urban, *Spine* **17** (1992) 1079.
59. R. Sah, A. Grodzinsky, A. Plaas and J. Sandy, in *Articular Cartilage and Osteoarthritis*, edited by K. Kuettner, R. Shleyerbach, J. Peyron and V. Hascall, (Raven Press, New York 1992) p.373.
60. J.P.G. Urban and A.S. Hall, *Ibid* p.393.
61. J.P.G. Urban, A.C. Hall and K.A. Gehl, *J. Cell. Physiol.* **154** (1993) 262.
62. M.L. Gray, A.M. Pizzanelli, A.J. Grodzinsky and R.C. Lee, *J. Orthop. Res.* **6** (1988) 777.
63. N. Boustany, M.L. Gray, A.C. Black and E.B. Hunziker, *J. Orthop. Res.* **in press** (1994)

64.   H.W. Jannasch, R.E. Marquis and A.M. Zimmerman, *Current perspectives in high pressure biology*, (Academic Press, London 1987).

65.   J.J. Parkkinen, M.J. Lammi, A. Pelttari, H.J. Helminen, M. Tammi and I. Virtanen, *Ann. Rheum. Dis.* **52** (1993) 192.

66.   S. Holm and J.P.G. Urban, in: *Joint Loading: biology and health of articular structures*, edited by H.J. Helminen, M. Tammi, I. Kiviranta, A.-M. Säämanen, K. Paukkonen and J. Jurvelin (Wright, Bristol, 1987) p.187.

67.   S. Holm, A. Maroudas, J. Urban, G. Selstam and A. Nachemson, *Connect. Tiss. Res.* **8** (1981) 101.

68.   H. Ishihara and J.P.G. Urban, *Trans. Am. Orthop. Res. Soc.*

69.   J.P.G. Urban, S. Holm and A. Maroudas, *Clin. Orthop.* **170** (1982) 293.

70.   B.P. O'Hara, J.P.G. Urban and A. Maroudas, *Ann. Rheum. Dis.* **49** (1990) 536.

CHAPTER 8

THE MICRO-ANATOMY OF INTERVERTEBRAL TISSUES IN THE NORMAL AND SCOLIOTIC SPINE

S. Roberts

1. Introduction

The functions of the spine, of weight bearing and movement, are directly dependent on the structure and organisation of its components. The cartilaginous tissues in the anterior region of the spine, the intervertebral disc and cartilage endplates (Figure 1), facilitate load bearing, and more particularly, bending of the spine in all directions. The manner in which these tissues are organised determines how they can function.

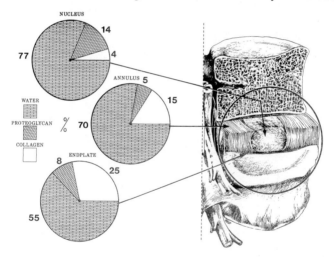

Figure 1. The location and composition of the cartilage endplate and intervertebral disc.

Histology allows us to study the structure at a microscopic level, which in turn gives rise to the macroscopic organisation. With the advent of poly- and monoclonal antibodies, immunolocalisation provides a method of determining the composition of a tissue in fine detail, both in the type of molecule present and its specific location within the tissue. Much work has and is being carried out in our department, utilising immunohistochemical techniques to define the organisation of both the intervertebral disc and cartilage endplate in normal and diseased states. Although scoliosis is more common in the thoracic spine, it also occurs in the lumbar spine, particularly in patients who present later in life. This chapter describes some recent findings concerning the micro-anatomy of the anterior intervertebral tissues in the normal spine and how this changes in scoliosis.

2. Gross anatomy

The intervertebral discs and cartilage endplates resemble other cartilages in that they are composed of a matrix consisting mainly of collagen fibres in a proteoglycan-water gel which is produced by cells within the tissues. The cartilage endplates are hyaline cartilage whilst the intervertebral disc is more akin to fibrocartilage. In the outer region of the disc, the annulus fibrosus, the matrix is arranged into a series of concentric rings.[14] Within adjacent rings the bundles of fibres change their line of orientation relative to the vertical, as can be seen in microscope sections viewed with polarised light (Figure 2). The central nucleus pulposus, in contrast, is less fibrous and the fibres that are present are more randomly arranged than in the annulus, particularly in young individuals.

The arrangement of collagen fibres and annular lamellae often differs in discs from patients with scoliosis compared to control material[28]. For example, severely crimped fibres, normally only found in the very outer annulus, are seen more within the annulus of some scoliotic patients. At the two opposite sides of the same scoliotic disc the annular lamellae often differed in their arrangement, either in number, size or orientation.

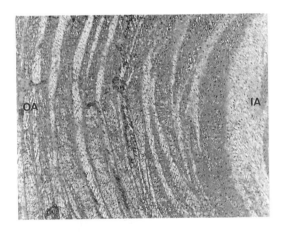

Figure 2. Section of disc viewed with polarised light demonstrating the organisation of the lamellar rings (4 year old human). These are narrower with more tightly packed collagen fibres towards the outer annulus (OA) than towards the inner (IA).

3. Matrix composition

Water is the main component of the disc and endplates. It is vital to the mechanical functioning of the tissues and is attracted there by the large, highly anionic proteoglycan molecules. These consist of a central protein core to which many side chains of glycosaminoglycans are attached, either keratan or chondroitin sulphate (Figure 3). It is these chains that confer the negative charges to the molecule, thus giving it the property to attract water and create a gel-like substance, so important to the functioning of the disc and cartilage. The amount of absorption of water, and swelling of the tissue, is restricted by the collagen fibres within the matrix. A review of the structure and function of the disc matrix can be found in Urban and Roberts[33].

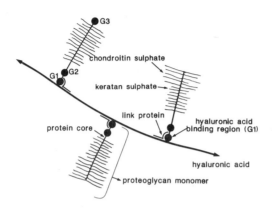

Figure 3. Structure of the most common proteoglycan in disc, aggrecan[33].

The composition of the matrix of both disc and cartilage endplate varies greatly with location in all directions (Figure 1)[29]. The regions closest to the central nucleus have the highest level of water and proteoglycan, but lowest collagen contents. There is a change in composition in both diseased and aged tissues, most notably a reduction in proteoglycan content, in comparison to young healthy tissue[23].

3.1. Collagen

Collagen is a family of at least 17 distinct proteins. They all have helical regions within the molecule, each type varying in the length and shape of the whole molecule and the proportion which is helical. The disc is composed of several collagen types, as summarised in Table 1. Types I and II collagen make up approximately 80% of the total collagen and form fibrils which provide the structural framework of the disc[7]. The outer annulus is predominantly type I, whilst the nucleus and cartilage endplates are predominantly type II. It is tempting to speculate that this reciprocal distribution is somehow related to the incident loading in the disc, since type I is predominant in other tissues with a high degree of tensile loading, for example tendon and ligament, and type II with a high level of compressive loading, for example articular cartilage.

Some collagen types, for example, III and VI occur mainly around the cells in normal human tissue and appear to form microfibrillar baskets or capsules around them, particularly in the nucleus (Figure 4)[27]. The function of these capsules remains unclear but suggestions for the presence in articular cartilage, at least, include a cell protecting role[16] or a mechanical role such as acting as a strain sensor enabling the cell to respond metabolically to a mechanical stimulus[5]. Alternatively, because type VI collagen has several RGD sequences, which are known to be involved in cell-matrix interactions in other tissues, the capsule could simply be a means of locating and binding the cell within the matrix.

Table 1. Collagen Types Found in the Intervertebral Disc

TYPE	LOCATION
I	Predominantly in outer annulus
	abundant in other tissues, eg tendon, bone[7]
II	Increasingly towards nucleus[7]
III	Mainly pericellular[27]
IV	Restricted to where blood vessels occur[27]
V	Annulus[7]
VI	Mainly pericellularly[7,27]
IX	Sometimes pericellularly[27]
X	Matrix and pericellularly[3]
XI	? predominantly nucleus, young endplate[7]

Although these minor collagen types account for only a small proportion of the total collagen, they may make a significant contribution to the overall functioning of the tissues. For example, in articular cartilage type IX collagen is cross-linked to type II collagen and appears to play a role in regulating the size of the type II fibres[34], which will have a direct effect on their mechanical functioning. The same is very likely true in intervertebral disc and cartilage endplates.

There is evidence that in scoliosis there may be a change in collagen synthesis and its distribution. For example, immunostaining for types III and VI collagens was greater in the matrix than round the cells in scoliotic individuals compared to that seen in non-scoliotic tissue. The distribution of type VI collagen, in particular, in scoliotic tissue resembles that of normal bovine disc rather than normal human discs[27]. Perhaps the increased presence within the matrix is a response to different loading in the bovine or scoliotic discs from that in normal human discs. Brickley-Parsons and Glimcher[4] also found a shift in both total collagen content and the ratio of types I:II collagen in discs from either side of the scoliotic spine, particularly at the apex of the curve. They suggest that the biological behaviour of the disc follows Wolff's Law in responding to the incident loading patterns.

3.2. Proteoglycans

It is becoming obvious that proteoglycans are also a family of molecules, varying in the size, type and length of glycosaminoglycan (GAG) chains present. The main proteoglycan in both disc and cartilage endplate is aggrecan, so called because individual molecules link together with others onto a chain of hyaluronic acid. This enables these molecules to form huge aggregates with molecular weights up to 2.6 million Da in articular cartilage. In intervertebral disc the proteoglycans are less aggregated and the

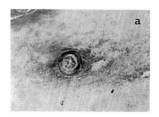 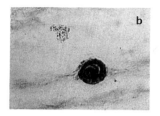

Figure 4. (a) Type III and (b) type VI collagen are preferentially stained around the cells of the human intervertebral disc.

monomers themselves are smaller, with shorter GAG chains and core proteins than in articular cartilage[10]. Following synthesis the aggrecans are converted to lower molecular weight forms by proteolytic degradation of the core protein. Recently another aggregating proteoglycan, versican, has been found to occur in small quantities in the disc, particularly the outer annulus[25]. This proteoglycan is typically produced by fibroblasts, which fits in with most staining in the matrix being seen in the outer annulus, where the cells are fibroblast-like.

Again immunolocalisation has demonstrated that the distribution of proteoglycans and various parts of the proteoglycan molecule is not homogenous throughout the matrix of the disc and cartilage endplate. More GAGs, particularly keratan sulphate, are found in the central nucleus pulposus than in the annulus. In adult tissues immunostaining is greater around the cells, in and within the capsular region[24]. In view of the steric interference and ionic effect that proteoglycans are known to have on the transport of large and charged substances respectively[33] this proteoglycan distribution may be very important to the cell activity allowing a molecular 'filtering' of substances towards and away from the cell.

The proteoglycan composition of some scoliotic discs and cartilage endplates has been shown to differ from normals[22]. For example, Melrose *et al.*[18] found more KS in discs from an individual with scoliosis than in similar aged cadaveric tissue.

3.3. Other macromolecules

Besides collagen and proteoglycan there are other macromolecules present in the intervertebral tissues, although details of them are often limited. These include elastin, fibrillin, amyloid and fibronectin, in addition to cytokines and enzymes and their inhibitors. There are other substances such as chondronectin or cartilage oligomeric matrix protein (COMP) which have been identified in allied cartilages, for example, articular cartilage, and may be found at a later date in the intervertebral cartilages.

Fibrillin is a glycoprotein which forms microfibrils and is involved in providing a framework for the deposition of elastin. It occurs in many tissues and is found to be abnormal in patients with Marfan's syndrome which has been linked to the fibrillin gene on chromosome 15[32]. Abnormal fibrillin has also been found in a small proportion of patients with idiopathic scoliosis[9]. Its presence in intervertebral disc and cartilage endplate is currently being investigated in our laboratory, particularly with regard to scoliosis.

4. Cell metabolism and maintenance of matrix

4.1. Cell types

The cells of the nucleus during foetal and infantile life are derived from the notochord. Using immunohistochemical markers for notochordal cells it has been shown that these cells are gradually replaced by chondrocytes, until after about 4 years of age, there are no notochordal cells remaining[21]. The chondrocytes are oval in shape and in adult discs lie either singly, or with increasing degeneration, in groups inside a fibrous capsule. In contrast, the cells of the annulus are narrow, elongated and may be desribed as fibroblast-like (Figure 5). They are aligned in the plane of the collagen bundles.

The density of cells in the intervertebral disc is very low[15] in comparison to other tissues, particularly in the nucleus. Their continuing activity is vital for the health and functioning of the disc, however, as the cells need to replace that matrix which breaks down and is lost with the passage of time.

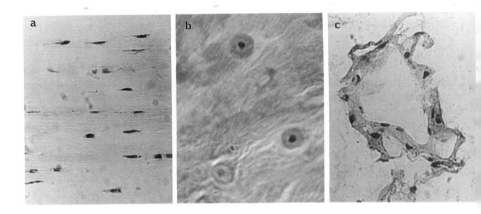

Figure 5. Cells of the human disc (a) annulus fibrosus, (b) nucleus pulposus and (c) notochordal cells.

4.2. Matrix synthesis

In-vitro studies on the metabolic activity of disc cells have demonstrated that these vary with location with the cells of the mid annulus generally having the highest rate of proteoglycan synthesis in the adult human intervertebral disc (Figure 6)[2].

Further studies have demonstrated that if the tissue is compressed, or loading reduced so that swelling can occur, then synthesis rates are greatly reduced[20]. Disc tissue from the concave side of the spine which is likely to be more compressed, has a lower GAG content, swelling pressure and water content than from the convex side[28,31]. This could be due to altered metabolic activity of the cells in reponse to different applied loads at each side. Immunolocalisation studies have demonstrated the presence of cells with a hyperactive morphology which produce type IX collagen, more commonly in scoliotic

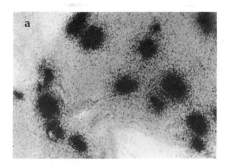 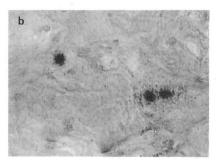

Figure 6. Autoradiography sections of human disc demonstrating greater uptake of radioactively labelled sulphate in (a) mid annulus than (b) nucleus.

tissue than in normal[21]. These same cells also stain for particular fragments of the proteoglycan molecule (unusually sulphated CS chains, expressing the 3B3- epitope),[30] which is typically seen either during growth and development or in some disease states.

4.3. Matrix degradation

The composition of any tissue is dependent, not only on how much is synthesised, but also on the rate of degradation of the matrix. Enzymes capable of breaking down the structural macromolecules of disc and cartilage matrix are known to occur in these tissues, including proteinases such as collagenase and stromolysin[19,14]. Inhibitors to many of them have also been indentified[17].

There is evidence suggesting that levels of these may be altered in diseases such as disc degeneration from those found at autopsy or scoliosis. Kang *et al.*[12] found that herniated discs had higher levels of gelatinase and stromolysin than those from scoliotic patients with no disc herniation. Recent studies indicate that different enzyme activities appear to exist at the compressed and uncompressed sides within the same scoliotic disc[6]. Most of the studies to date have utilised biochemical methods or zymography and hence give no indication of the location of these enzymes and their inhibitors. Immunolocalisation studies are underway to determine whether their expression is restricted to certain localities, eg histologically degenerate areas.

5. Nutrition and vascularisation

In the adult, the intervertebral disc and cartilage endplate are normally avascular and as such rely on the diffusion of solutes from the blood supply of adjacent tissues for their cellular nutrition. These are mainly the vertebral body and the longitudinal ligaments.

In young individuals, such as many of those with idiopathic scoliosis, and in people with disc degeneration the discs can be quite highly vascularised, at least in the outer and mid annulus. This can be visualised using antibodies to endothelial markers (Figure 7).

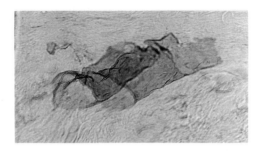

Figure 7. Section of disc stained with antibodies to an endothelial marker, demonstrating blood vessels in the annulus of a patient with scoliosis.

6. Innervation and neuropeptide distribution

Innervation of the intervertebral disc occurs in the outer annulus fibrosus (Figure 8) and the adjacent longitudinal ligaments[1,35]. Some of the nerves are immunoreactive to calcitonin gene related peptide (CGRP), substance P (SP) and vasoactive intestinal peptide (VIP), neuropeptides which may participate in sensory transmission[1]. There is, however, no clear evidence of the innervation extending into either the nucleus pulposus or the cartilage endplate[26].

An immunolocalisation investigation into the distribution of nerves and neuropeptides in disc tissue from different localities within the spine of scoliotic patients has recently been undertaken[26]. Surgical specimens were carefully dissected so that material from opposite sides of the curve could be compared. There was a difference in degree of staining in 23 of 36 such pairs of samples, with most having a greater innervation towards the uncompressed region than the compressed region, although numbers were too small to prove statistical significance. It was suspected that since some of the neuropeptides can affect the metabolism of connective tissue cells, this uneven distribution could be a reason for the asymmetrical growth seen in scoliosis.

7. Calcification

Calcium deposits in intervertebral discs have been reported previously and identified as either calcium pyrophosphate dihydrate or hydroxyapatite[8]. More recently a histological study has demonstrated calcification of cartilage endplates from patients of all ages with scoliosis[28]. The calcium salts were identified as poorly organised calcium hydroxyapatite. The degree of calcification varied, ranging from deposits on or around a few cells to extensive blocks of calcification through the cartilage endplate (Figure 9). Sometimes ossification within the calcified region occurred, with clear osseous lamellae present. Calcification occasionally extended into the intervertebral disc but never occurred in the disc alone. As most patients with scoliosis, particularly idiopathic, are first seen

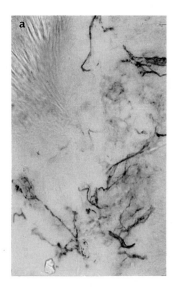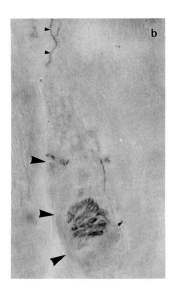

Figure 8. Section of human disc, stained with a general nerve marker, antibodies to protein gene product (PGP), demonstrating (a) a nerve plexus in the annulus fibrosus and (b) a sensory nerve ending, a mechanoreceptor (large arrows), with the nerve possibly leading to it (small arrows).

before they have reached skeletal maturity, endochondral ossification should be ongoing in epiphysial regions such as the cartilage endplate. Calcification in this location is therefore likely to affect growth, either by acting as a tether and, or affecting the nutrition of the endplate. It could also be expected to affect the loading of the tissues since calcification stiffens the matrices. In addition, since the adult disc is avascular, it relies on diffusion of substances to and from the vasculature within adjacent tissues for the provision of nutrients and clearance of waste products. One of these pathways is from the vertebral body via the cartilage endplate. Calcification here could therefore be expected to affect the rate of transport of solutes through it and so may decrease the nutritive flow to the disc.

8. Summary of changes in the scoliotic spine

8.1. Collagen

The type of collagen present, the quantity and the gross organisation of it all appear to be affected in scoliosis. There is a difference in these properties in intervertebral tissues from the concave side of the curve compared to the convex side, with the most difference often being found at the apex of the curve. Alteration of the collagen makeup will obviously have far reaching effects on the flexibility and mechanical properties of the disc, since these are dependent on the organisation of the collagen fibrils.

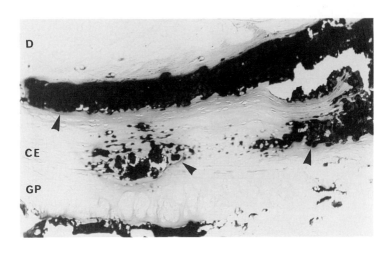

Figure 9. Section from 12 year old boy with scoliosis, stained with von Kossa, demonstrating extensive calcification (arrows) in the region of the cartilage endplate (CE). (D: Disc, GP: growth plate.)

8.2. Proteoglycan and water

The quantity of total proteoglycan and water also differs between regions of the scoliotic spine, together with the type of glycosaminoglycan present. Since the amount of distension of collagen fibres depends on the swelling caused by the proteoglycans, a change in the amount or type of this could also be expected to affect the mechanical properties, particularly the handling of compressive loads.

8.3. Neuropeptides

Preliminary results indicate a difference in the degree of innervation, with more innervation apparent towards the uncompressed compared to the compressed region in many scoliotic discs. Since some neuropeptides can influence the metabolism of connective tissue cells, this could be a mechanism for the asymmetrical growth seen in scoliosis.

8.4. Calcification

Deposition of calcium hydroxyapatite crystals is a common occurrence in the cartilage endplate of scoliotic patients, regardless of age of onset or type of scoliosis. This could be expected to affect, not only the mechanical response of the tissue to loading, but also growth of the vertebral segment and, since one of the main nutritive pathways to disc is via the endplate, the metabolism of the cells of the intervertebral disc. It is very likely that calcification in this location is directly related to the rigidity of the curve.

It is clear that many differences in properties occur both between scoliotic and non-scoliotic disc and cartilage endplate and also at varying locations within the scoliotic spine. What is not clear, however, is whether these are primary or secondary effects. It is to be expected that many are a secondary response to altered loading within the scoliotic spine. Even if this is the case, they may still be of paramount importance to the development of the scoliosis and hence the management of the disorder.

9. Acknowledgements

Financial assistance for much of the work described in this chapter has been provided by the Arthritis and Rheumatism Council, the Stanley Watson Barker Trust and the JR Levy Scholarship via the British Scoliosis Society.

10. References

1. I.K. Ashton, S. Roberts, D.C. Jaffray, J.M. Polak and S.M. Eisenstein, *J. Orthop. Res.* **12** (1994) 186-192.
2. M.T. Bayliss, B. Johnstone and J.P. O'Brien, *Spine* **13** (1988) 972-981.
3. N. Boos, A. Nerlich, K. Von Der Mark, and M. Aeb, *Trans. Am. Orthop. Res.* **19** (1994)
4. D. Brickley-Parsons and M.J. Glimcher, *Spine* **9** (1984) 148-163.
5. N.D. Broom and D.B. Myers, *Connect. Tissue Res.* **7** (1980) 227- 237.
6. J. Crean, V.C. Duance and S. Roberts, unpublished data.
7. D.R. Eyre, in *The biology of the intervertebral disc*, ed. P. Ghosh (CRC Press Inc., Boca Raton, 1988).
8. J. Feinberg, O. Boachie-Adjei, O.P.G. Bullough, A.L. Boskey, *Clin. Orthop. Res.* **254** (1990) 303-310.
9. N. Hadley-Miller, B. Mims and D.M. Milewicz, *J. Bone Joint Surg.* **76A** (1994) 1193-1206.
10. B. Johnstone and M.T. Bayliss, *Spine* (1994) In press.
11. B. Johnstone, M. Markopoulos, P. Neame and B. Caterson, *Biochem. J.* **292** (1993) 661-666.
12. J.D. Kang, H.I. Georgescu, L. McIntyr, M. Stefanovic-Racic, I. Nita, W.F. Donaldson and C.H. Evans, *Procs ISSLS* (1994) 11
13. J. Liu, P.J. Roughley and J.S. Mort, *J. Orthop. Res.* **9** (1991) 568-575.
14. F. Marchand and A.M. Ahmed, *Spine* **15** (1990) 402-410.
15. A. Maroudas, R.A. Stockwell, A. Nachemson and J.P.G. Urban, *J. Anat.* **120** (1975) 113-130.
16. G. Meachim and R.A. Stockwell, in *Adult Articular Cartilage*, ed. M.A.R. Freeman (Pitman Medical, Bath, 1979).
17. J. Melrose, P. Ghosh and T.K.F. Taylor, *Matrix* **12** (1992) 56-75.
18. J. Melrose, K.R.Gurr, T-C. Cole, A. Darvodelsky, P. Ghosh and T.K.F. Taylor, *J. Orthop. Res.* **9** (1991) 68-77.

19.   S.C. Ng, J.B. Weiss, R. Quennel and M.I.V. Jayson, *Spine* **11** (1986) 695-701.

20.   H. Oshima, J.P.G. Urban and D.H. Bergel, *J. Orthop. Res.* (1994) In press.

21.   U.E. Pazzaglia, J.R. Salisbury and P.D. Byers, *J. Royal Soc. Med.* **82** (1989) 413-415.

22.   A. Pedrini-Mille, V.A. Pedrini, C. Tusimo, I.V. Ponseti, S.L. Weinstein and J.A. Maynard, *J. Bone Joint Surg.* **65A** (1983) 815-823.

23.   S. Roberts, H.K. Beard and J.P. O'Brien, *Annals of Rheumatic Diseases,* **41** (1982) 78-85.

24.   S. Roberts, B. Caterson, H. Evans and S.M. Eisenstein, *Histochem. J.* **26** (1994a) 402-411.

25.   S. Roberts, B. Johnstone, H. Evans and S.M. Eisenstein, *Int. J. Exp. Pathol.* (1993a).

26.   S. Roberts, J. Menage, K. Ashton and S. Eisenstein, *J. Bone Joint Surg.* (1994b) In press.

27.   S. Roberts, J. Menage, V. Duance, S. Wotton and S. Ayad, *Spine* **16** (1991) 1030-1038.

28.   S. Roberts, J. Menage and S.M. Eisenstein, *J. Orthop. Res.* **11** (1993b) 747-757.

29.   S. Roberts, J. Menage and J.P. Urban, *Spine* **14** (1989) 166-174.

30.   S. Roberts and B Caterson. unpublished data

31.   C. Tighe, J.C.T. Fairbanks and J.P.G. Urban, *J. Bone Joint Surg.* (1994) In press

32.   P. Tsipouras, R.D. Mastro, M. Sarfarazi, B. Lee, E. Vitale, A.C. Child, *et al*, *New Eng. J.* **326** (1992) 905-909.

33.   J.P.G. Urban and S. Roberts, in *Grieve's Modern Manual Therapy of the Vertebral Column, eds Boyling and Palastanga* (Churchill Livingsone, Edinburgh, 1994).

34.   S. Wotton, V.C. Duance and P.R. Fryer, *FEBS Lett.* **23** (1988) 79-82.

35.   H. Yoshizawa, J.P. o'Brien, W.T. Smith and M Trumper, *J. Pathol.* **132** (1980) 95-104.

CHAPTER 9

NEUROPEPTIDES IN THE LUMBAR SPINE

I.K. Ashton and S.M. Eisenstein

1. Introduction

Back pain is prevalent in adult western populations to the extent that it is regarded as integral to the human condition. The proportion of the population suffering chronic debilitating pain consumes enormous medical and financial resources for disappointingly little benefit. No matter how social, cultural and psychological factors may modify the perception of pain and pain-related disability, there can be no hope of coming closer to an improved treatment for chronic back pain without an understanding of pain chemistry and anatomy.

One approach to the better understanding of the origins of back pain has been prompted by the principle that a tissue can evoke pain only if it has a nerve supply. This has led to numerous investigations into the neural anatomy of the lumbar spine.

Widespread innervation has been revealed in most of the structures of the spine, i.e. the facet capsule, the annulus fibrosus of the intervertebral disc, the adjacent anterior and posterior longitudinal ligaments, the supraspinous and interspinous ligaments, the periosteum and marrow of the vertebral body and the spinal muscles. However, not all the innervation revealed by traditional histological methods is sensory or nociceptive nor do these methods always reveal the fine non-myelinated nerve fibres.

Nociceptors are the neural sensors which signal harmful or potentially harmful stimuli to the central nervous system and are considered to have a protective function. The afferent fibres of nociceptors are found amongst the thinly myelinated $A\delta$ or nonmyelinated C-fibres which terminate in the spinal cord. These are mainly high threshold, slowly conducting (Group III and IV) fibres which are normally activated only by noxious stimuli. This is in contrast to the low threshold, fast conducting (Group I and II) fibres which, in the normal situation, are activated by innocuous stimuli such as gentle pressure or normal movement.

Recently, specific immunohistochemical techniques have enabled fine afferent nerve fibres to be more readily demonstrated in tissue sections. It has also been possible to identify the neuropeptide content of these nerves. This chapter describes several of these studies and outlines the possible roles of the neuropeptides in the lumbar spine.

1.1. Neuropeptides

Many neuropeptides are produced in the cell bodies of the primary afferent neurons within the dorsal root ganglia. These include substance P, calcitonin gene related peptide, vasoactive intestinal peptide, dynorphin, galanin, enkephalin, somatostatin and cholecystokinin, the first three of which, together with neuropeptide Y, will be discussed in this chapter.

Substance P is an 11 amino acid peptide which has been localized in small diameter, unmyelinated, C-type primary afferents representing approximately a third of the C-fibre population at most spinal levels. Because of its localization and other features it has been implicated in nociception and vasoactivity.

Calcitonin gene related peptide (CGRP) is a 37 amino acid product of alternative splicing of the calcitonin gene. CGRP co-localizes with substance P in C-fibres but is also found in the thinly myelinated Ad fibres and motor nerves. CGRP can promote nociception by potentiating substance P release and the two peptides can act synergistically to modulate nociceptive responses. CGRP is a potent vasodilator and may have a co-regulatory vasomotor function with substance P.

Vasoactive intestinal peptide (VIP) is a 28 amino acid peptide with widespread neuronal localization. In addition to fulfilling many of the criteria of a sensory neurotransmitter, VIP also regulates a number of autonomic events e.g. blood flow.
On activation of afferent fibres, neuropeptides are delivered by axonal transport to sites of release in the central nervous system and, as will be described later, to peripheral tissues. The afferent fibres have their synaptic contacts in the substantial gelatinosa of the dorsal horn. Synaptic transmission of nociceptive messages is thought to depend on excitatory amino acids e.g. glutamate and neuropeptides such as substance P, CGRP and VIP which cooperate to excite the dorsal horn neurons. These then relay information to spinal motor and autonomic nerves and to the ascending pathways to the brain.
Although pain is classically regarded as being mediated solely by the sensory neurons, the autonomic nervous system and its transmitters are increasingly thought to be involved in pain syndromes[1]. Neuropeptide Y, a 36 amino acid peptide, is widely distributed in sympathetic neurons. Its coexistence with noradrenaline suggests its role in autonomic transmission. In contrast to the previously described peptides, neuropeptide Y is a potent vasoconstrictor.
In order to achieve a better understanding of neurological processes in the lumbar spine we have investigated the distribution of these peptides in a variety of spinal tissues.

2. Localization of neuropeptides in spinal tissue

2.1. Demonstration of neuropeptides by immunohistochemistry.
Spinal tissue for analysis was fixed in Zamboni's fluid for 4-24 h as soon as possible after removal then washed with 0.1 M phosphate buffered saline containing 15%(w/v) sucrose[2]. The tissue was frozen in Arcton 12 or isopentane and mounted on cork blocks such that 10-30 μm cryostat sections could be obtained. The sections were treated with 3% hydrogen peroxide to quench endogenous peroxidase activity then incubated in buffer containing polyclonal antisera to substance P, CGRP, VIP or the C-peptide of neuropeptide Y at appropriate dilutions. This was followed by incubation with biotinylated goat anti-rabbit IgG and the avidin biotin reagent (ABC). Peroxidase reaction product was enhanced with the glucose oxidase nickel diaminobenzidine method. Immunostaining was absent in sections from which the primary antisera had been withheld or replaced with non-immune rabbit serum.

2.2. Facet capsule

The facet joint capsule consists of an outer layer of fibroelastic connective tissue, a middle vascular, fatty layer and an inner synovial lining membrane. The fibrous capsule of the joint is well innervated, receiving a nerve supply from the medial branches of at least two consecutive posterior primary rami.

In our study we have examined this innervation more closely in facet capsule removed during spinal fusion for degenerate disc disease or facet arthrosis[2]. Immunohistochemical staining of facet capsule revealed abundant, fine (<2 mm) CGRP immunoreactive fibres in the fibrous and adipose layers (Figure 1). Approximately half of the fibres were localized perivascularly. Nerves immunoreactive for VIP were also present in the facet capsule, always running freely in the tissue stroma, never in association with blood vessels. We also demonstrated sparse substance P immunoreactivity in the facet capsule. Neuropeptide Y (identified by its C-peptide) was the most abundant of the neuropeptides in the facet capsule (Figure 2). Neuropeptide Y immunoreactive nerves were invariably found in close proximity to blood vessels, frequently encircling them.

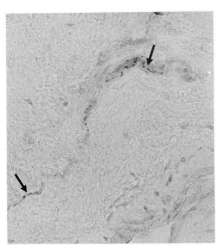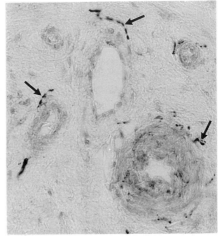

Figure 1   Figure 2

Substance P containing nerves have also been described in the inferior recess capsule and synovial folds of the lumbosacral joint[3]. These authors suggested that the nerve fibres may cause pain if the synovial fold impinges between the zygapophyseal facets. Others have confirmed the presence of substance P immunoreactive nerves surrounding blood vessels and in plical synovial tissue. Similarly, a small number of substance P immunoreactive fibres were demonstrated in the facet capsule of the rabbit by an indirect immunofluorescence technique[4].

The consensus of these studies is that substance P and CGRP immunoreactive nerves account for a relatively small proportion of the total innervation of the facet capsule.

Electrophysiological studies have indicated the presence of slowly adapting nerve fibres which can be stimulated by substance P in the rat facet capsule. Taken together the data suggest the presence in facet capsule of nociceptive fibres which could be important in pain production caused by excessive load or stretch or by chemical mediators.

Degenerative disease in the facet capsule affects subchondral bone as well as the capsule. In degenerate facet joints, substance P immunoreactive nerves were found in erosion channels which extended from the subchondral bone into the articular cartilage and also in the marrow spaces[5]. Substance P fibres were usually seen in proximity to small blood vessels coursing from the subchondral bone to the 'tidemark'. The similarity of this innervation with that of the patella in degenerative arthritis, in which the histological findings are similar[6], suggests a similar process of degenerative change.

The ventral aspect of the facet capsule extends into the ligamentum flavum. Although the superficial layer is innervated, we and others have found no neuropeptide imunoreactive nerves in ligamentum flavum[2].

2.3. Ligaments

The sinuvertebral nerve, which contains both a sensory and a sympathetic component, innervates the ligamentous structures of the lumbar spine. Neural elements have been shown to be especially abundant in the posterior longitudinal ligaments obtained during surgery for disc herniations[7]. Both substance P and CGRP immunoreactive nerves were evident and serial sections showed that the peptides could be localized in the same nerve fibres. The nerve fibres were described as being usually unrelated to blood vessels although occasionally in direct apposition to small blood vessels.

In studies of the rat lumbar spine, fine, varicose, substance P and CGRP immunoreactive fibres were found in both the anterior and the posterior longitudinal ligaments with the posterior longitudinal ligament being most densely innervated[8]. Perivascular CGRP immunoreactive fibres were found whereas substance P immunoreactive fibres were usually not by blood vessels. A similar distribution was found in the interspinous ligament. Substance P immunoreactive fibres were also found in the supraspinous ligament of the rabbit. It has been suggested that the presence of these sensory nerves in ligaments may account for pain perceived if pressure is applied to ligaments by spondylophytes[9].

Both neuropeptide Y and VIP immunoreactive fibres were more numerous in the posterior longitudinal ligament than in the anterior longitudinal ligament of the rabbit. Neuropeptide Y was predominantly located near blood vessels in contrast to VIP immunoreactive nerves which were mostly not associated with the vasculature.

2.4. Intervertebral disc

The sinuvertebral nerve and the grey ramus communicantes terminate in the intervertebral disc. The presence of nerve fibres in the superficial layers of the disc, penetrating the outer third at least of the annulus fibrosus, have been described in man and other species.

We have further investigated the nature of the innervation by immuno-histochemical demonstration of several neuropeptides in intervertebral disc obtained during anterior fusion for back pain or corrective surgery for scoliosis.[10,11] Nerve fibres immunoreactive for CGRP were clearly demonstrated (Figure 3), some of them, but not all, being in the vicinity of blood vessels. This was in accord with a similar distribution of CGRP fibres in the outer layers of the annulus fibrosus which has been described in the rat[12]. We have also identified substance P immunoreactive nerves (Figure 4) in the anterior, posterior and lateral parts of the disc, also in the outer annulus. Rarely, these fibres were found in the vicinity of blood vessels (Figure 5). As we have found in other tissues and as other investigators have reported, substance P immunoreactive fibres are very difficult to identify. The fibres are very fine, often only faintly stained and can be clearly observed only by continuous readjustment of the fine focus of the microscope through the depth of the tissue section. Profuse nerve fibres immunoreactive for VIP were clearly seen running circumferentially in the annulus fibrosus (Figure 6). As in the facet capsule, VIP fibres were not related to blood vessels.

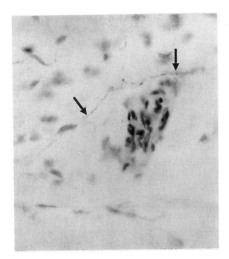
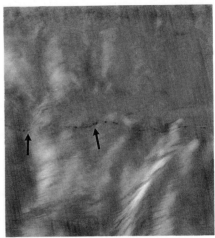

Figure 3   Figure 4

It has long been known that the intervertebral disc could be painful to palpation under local anaesthetic. The demonstration of CGRP, VIP and substance P immunoreactive fibres in the annulus fibrosus indicates a sensory innervation that could be susceptible to stimulation by raised intradiscal pressure or chemical mediators resulting from disc damage or degeneration.

Immunoreactivity to neuropeptide Y was localized exclusively close to blood vessels[10]. Neuropeptide Y has also been demonstrated in the vascular channels of the bony endplate of the disc and may be involved in the regulation of blood flow and hence nutrition of the intervertebral disc[13].

Innervation has only rarely been reported in the nucleus pulposus and this has been in degenerate discs. We have not found neuropeptide innervation in the nucleus pulposus even though many of the discs were degenerate.

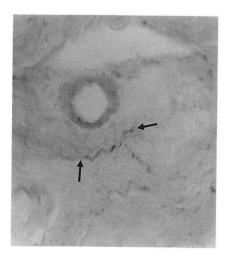 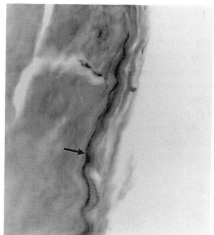

Figure 5

Figure 6

2.5. Bone

Nerve fibres from the sympathetic trunk and the grey ramus communicantes as well as plexuses from the longitudinal ligaments, penetrate the vertebral body. VIP immunoreactive fibres were localized in the periosteum of porcine[14] and rat[15] vertebral body. VIP fibres were found in the bone marrow appearing as long varicose terminals mostly unrelated to blood vessels. Numerous VIP fibres were also found at the osteochondral junction of the vertebral growth plate. The predominantly nonvascular distribution of the fibres in the vertebral body suggests that the role of VIP in bone is not primarily vasoregulatory as it is in other tissues. Interestingly, VIP administration did not affect blood flow in bone[14]. Instead the major role of VIP in the bone may relate to bone cell physiology.

Thin, varicose, substance P immunoreactive fibres were also observed, primarily in bone marrow not usually close to blood vessels[8]. In contrast, CGRP fibres were commonly perivascular. Both substance P and CGRP were found close to the growth plate. No immunoreactivity for either VIP, substance P or CGRP has been identified in cortical bone of the verebral body.

Neuropeptide Y immunoreactive fibres were found in the vertebral body and periosteum of rat lumbar spine[15]. These fibres were particularly abundant in the bone marrow and the vertebral growth plate, the majority being close to or within the vessel wall.

2.6. The spondylolysis 'ligament'

The defect in the pars interarticularis of the posterior neural arch in spondylolysis is bridged by tissue which has been described as ligamentous. We have confirmed the ligamentous nature of the tissue[16]. Histology revealed parallel linearity of collagen fibres directed between the bone insertions.

Immunohistochemical methods showed the presence of nerve fibres surrounding the ligament especially around the adipose tissue and also in the ligament itself. CGRP immunoreactive fibres were found amongst blood vessels and between fat cells. Occasionally fine, varicose, CGRP fibres were also found in the ligament (Figure 7) as were fibres immunoreactive to VIP. Some of the VIP fibres were perivascular which is of interest as this has not been the case in other spinal tissues such as facet capsule or disc. Many of the nerve fibres in the associated vascular tissue were immunoreactive to neuropeptide Y (Figure 8).

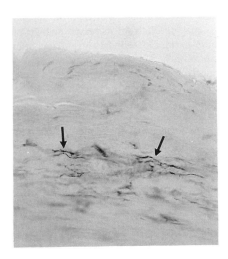 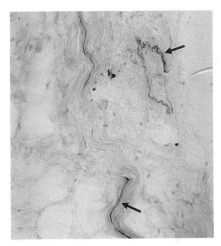

Figure 7   Figure 8

The extent of innervation of the spondylolysis ligament varied among patients and this may reflect the duration of the defect or the degree of organization of the ligament. In any event the presence of neural elements in and around the structure could constitute an additional source of pain in patients with low back pain in the presence of spondylolysis.

3. Implications for nociception

The immunohistochemical studies which have been described have demonstrated the widespread occurrence of the neuropeptides substance P, CGRP, VIP and neuropeptide Y in most structures of the lumbar spine, with the notable exception of the ligamentum flavum and the nucleus pulposus of the intervertebral disc. While some variation may be due to the technical differences associated with fixation and handling of the various tissues and the sensitivities of the antisera, similar data has now been presented in tissue obtained from both animals and man.

Interestingly, the tissues in which innervation has been demonstrated are those in which pain can be evoked by pressure, injection of isotonic saline or other means of stimulation. In contrast, ligamentum flavum, and the nucleus pulposus appear to be insensitive to surgical procedures in which annulus fibrosus and vertebral endplate are particularly sensitive[17].

Similar neuropeptide innervation has been described in tissues from normal animals and in surgical specimens obtained from procedures either for deformity (scoliosis) or back pain. No relationship has been demonstrated between the extent of innervation and back pain or disc degeneration in any of the studies. Indeed, interpretation of quantitative data might be difficult. For example, in arthritic synovium and bone marrow the apparent paucity of substance P immunoreactive nerves may result from increased endogenous proteolysis of the peptide in the peripheral nerve terminals secondary to inflammation, rather than from the absence of the nerves themselves[18].

Despite these limitations, there is clear evidence that normal and pathological tissues of the lumbar spine have sensory nerve fibres which contain substance P, VIP and CGRP. Evidence from many sources suggests that such fibres are nociceptive and that the peptides play a key role in the transmission of nociceptive information in the central nervous system. The actual interactive processes involved are currently the focus of much research. The noxious events which might excite the nociceptors in the lumbar spine could be excessive compression or abnormal stretch of the capsule of ligaments. Pain elicited in this way is likely to be of short duration. However, even brief activation of nociceptive C-fibres increases the response of spinal neurons to sensory inputs which result in the normally low threshold mechanoreceptors beginning to elicit pain[19]. The duration of the perceived pain is thus amplified many fold.

As is readily observed in orthopaedic practice, pain can be elicited by stimuli which are normally regarded as innocuous. Abnormal sensitivity of the sensory nervous system due to reduction in the normally high threshold of nociceptive afferents may result from repeated noxious stimuli, nerve damage, ischaemia or chemical mediators eg. bradykinin, prostaglandin, leukotrienes etc. released by inflammatory processes[20]. Cytokines released by inflammatory cells can also upregulate the synthesis of substance P and CGRP in the dorsal root ganglia with subsequent amplification of afferent input to the spinal cord .

Almost all of the spinal tissues examined contained neuropeptide Y immunoreactive nerves. Neuropeptide Y is indicative of sympathetic innervation but this may have implications for pain perception because of the interaction between the sympathetic and sensory nervous systems[1].

4. Peripheral functions of neuropeptides

Apart from their sensory nociceptive function, somatosensory C-fibres have a neurosecretory role. In response to mechanical and chemical stimuli, a substantial proportion of the neuropeptides which are synthesized in the dorsal root ganglia are transported to the peripheral nerve terminals. Our studies and those of others have described the substance P and CGRP immunoreactive nerves in the lumbar spine as varicose. These varicosities represent the synaptic vesicles of nerve terminals where the processing of the neuropeptides is completed and from which they are released.

The concentrations of neuropeptides in peripheral tissues, including in rat knees, has been measured[21]. Since substance P, CGRP and VIP may be released into the 'tissues of the spine, the possible local effects of the neuropeptides on spinal tissues should be considered.

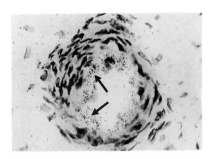

Figure 9

4.1. Blood flow and inflammation

CGRP immunoreactive nerves have been clearly identified adjacent to blood vessels in facet capsule, ligaments, intervertebral disc and bone. CGRP is a potent vasodilator and may participate in vasomotor control as well as in nociception. Although substance P containing nerves have been less frequently associated with blood vessels in the lumbar spine than CGRP, substance P is also known to increase plasma extravasation and vasodilation. In synovium, for example, substance P interacts with specific neurokinin type 1 (NK1) receptors located on endothelial cells of blood vessels which leads to the release of the endothelial cell relaxing factor, nitric oxide. In our search for possible substance P receptors in the intervertebral disc we have identified NK1 receptors on endothelial cells of small blood vessels in the outer annulus fibrosus (Figure 9) by autoradiography using ^{125}I-substance P[22]. We have suggested that substance P may therefore have similar vasoactive and inflammatory effects in intervertebral disc as it has in synovium.

Substance P has other pro-inflammatory effects such as stimulating mast cell degranulation and histamine release, lymphocyte proliferation, the promotion of free radical release from neutrophils and the induction of IL1 and TNF α from macrophages.

Substance P, CGRP and VIP have considerable functional relationship, in particular, synergistic or potentiating effects on vasoactivity and inflammatory responses. It is therefore of interest that the peptides appear to occur in the majority of spinal tissues studied and in some, co-localization of substance P and CGRP in the same nerve fibre has been indicated.

Neuropeptide Y has been found exclusively in association with blood vessels in all the studies of spinal tissues. The distribution of neuropeptide Y and the reported effect of sympathetic denervation in increasing blood flow suggest that an important function of neuropeptide Y in the spine, particularly in bone marrow and the bony endplate may be vasoregulatory.

VIP, although a known vasoactive peptide in many tissues, was not found in association with blood vessels in the spine except in the spondylolysis ligament so is unlikely to have a significant vasoactive role. Instead, VIP may, together with CGRP, modify immune function. In contrast to substance P, CGRP and VIP suppress lymphocyte proliferation and macrophage activation.

4.2. Tissue effects

Substance P is a cell mitogen, stimulating fibroblast and synoviocyte proliferation and endothelial cell migration. In inflammatory synovium, substance P may contribute to angiogenesis and in view of our demonstration of substance P receptors on endothelial cells in the intervertebral disc we have suggested that substance P might be involved in the neovascularization seen in some degenerate discs. We have also reported that substance P has stimulatory effects on proliferation and proteoglycan synthesis in rabbit intervertebral disc cells in culture[23]. Whether these effects are physiologically relevant to the metabolism of mature human disc remains to be investigated.

CGRP also stimulates fibroblast proliferation and this, together with its vasoactive effects, has suggested that CGRP may have a role in tissue repair and the proper orientation of collagen fibres in healing ligament[24]. The presence of substance P, CGRP and neuropeptide Y immunoreactive nerves in the chondroblastic fibrous tissue in a bone induction model[25] and the extension of CGRP immunoreactive fibres into small erosions in the joints of arthritic rats have also been interpreted as contributions to tissue repair.[18]

Neuroendocrine regulation of bone cell metabolism has been demonstrated with CGRP, VIP, substance P or neuropeptide Y in a variety of osteoblastic cell cultures and in human bone marrow stromal cells *in vitro*[26]. *In vitro*, VIP also stimulates bone resorption[14] while CGRP appears to have the opposite effect. Substance P can stimulate bone resorption through enhanced IL1 and TNF α production, and fibroblast-mediated prostaglandin release. The nervous system may therefore contribute to bone remodelling by increased neuropeptide synthesis and peripheral release in response to injury or inflammation.

5. Conclusion

The field of neuropeptide research is moving ahead rapidly. With the potential for selective anti-nociceptive agents and more specifically targeted anti-inflammatory therapies[27], some of which are now in the process of clinical trials, a detailed understanding of the neural anatomy of the lumbar spine has obvious importance. Whether the neuropeptides contribute to connective tissue metabolism, tissue repair or bone remodelling and whether this could be therapeutically exploited remains to be established.

6. References

1. J.D. Levine, S.J. Dardick, M.F. Roizen, C. Helms and A.I. Basbaum, *J. Neurosciences* **6** (1986) 3423-2429.
2. I.K. Ashton, B.A. Ashton, S.J. Gibson, J.M. Polak, D.C. Jaffray and S.M. Eisenstein, *J. Orthop. Res.* **10** (1992) 72-78.
3. L.G.F. Giles and A.R. Harvey, *Br. J. Rheumatol* **26** (1987), 362-364.
4. A. El-Bohy, J.M. Cavanaugh, M.L. Getchell, T. Bulas, T.V. Getchell and A King, *Brain Research* **460** (1988) 379-382.
5. D.N. Beaman, G.P. Graziano, R.A. Glover, E.M. Wojtys and V. Chang, *Spine* **18** (1993) 1044-1049.
6. S.M. Eisenstein and C.R. Parry, *J. Bone Joint Surg.* **69-B** (1987) 3-7.
7. Y.T. Konttinen, M. Gronblad, I. Antti-Poika, S. Seitsalo, S. Santavirta, M. Hukkanen and J.M. Polak, *Spine* **15** (1990) 383-386.
8. M. Ahmed, A. Bjurholm, A. Kreicbergs and M. Schultzberg, *Neuro Orthopedics* **12** (1991) 19-28.
9. B. Vernon-Roberts, in *The lumbar spine and back pain*, ed. M.I.V. Jayson (Pitman Medical, UK, 1980) 83-114.
10. I.K. Ashton, S. Roberts, D.C. Jaffray, J.M. Polak and S.M. Eisenstein, *J. Orthop. Res.* **12** (1994) 186-192.
11. I.K .Ashton, D.A. Walsh, S. Roberts, J.M. Polak and S.M. Eisenstein, *J. Bone Joint S.* **76-B** (1994) supp 1.
12. P.W. McCarthy, B. Carruthers, D. Martin and P. Petts, *Spine* **16** (1991) 653-655.
13. M. Brown, M. Hukkanen, H. Crock, T. Shirashi, J. Polak and S. Hughes. Presented at the Society for Back Pain Research, London, October 1992.
14. E.L. Hohmann, R.P. Elde, J.A. Rysavy, S. Einzig and R.L. Gebhard, *Science* **223** (1986) 868-871.
15. M. Ahmed, A.Bjurholm, A.Kreicbergs and M. Schultzberg, *Spine* **18** (1993) 268- 273.
16. S.M. Eisenstein, I.K. Ashton, S. Roberts, A.J. Darby, P. Kanse, J. Menage and H. Evans, *Spine* **19** (1994) 912-916.
17. S.D. Kuslich, J.W. Ahern and D.L. Tarr. Presented at the Lumbar Spine Symposium, Brussels, August 1994.
18. M. Hukkanen, Y.T. Konttinen, R.G. Rees, S.J. Gibson, S. Santavirta and J.M. Polak, *J. Rheumatol.* **19** (1992) 1252-1259.
19. C.J. Woolf, *Brit. Med. Bull.* **47** (1991) 523-533.
20. H.-G. Schaible, and R.F. Schmidt, *J. Neurophysiol.* **54** (1985), 1109-1122.
21. M. Ahmed, A, Bjurholm, G.R. Srinivasan, E. Theodorsson and A. Kreicbergs, *Peptides* **15** (1994) 317-322.
22. I.K. Ashton, D.A. Walsh, J.M. Polak, S.M. Eisenstein, *Acta Orthop. Scand.* **65** (1994) In Press.
23. I.K. Ashton, G.L. Risley, R. Prue and S. M. Eisenstein, Presented at the Lumbar Spine Symposium, Brussels, August 1994.

24.   M. Gronblad, O. Korkala, Y.T. Konttinen, H. Kuokkanen and P. Liesi, *Clin Orthop.* **265** (1991) 291-295.

25.   A. Bjurholm, A. Kreicbergs, L. Dahlberg and M. Schultzberg, *Bone and Mineral* **10** (1990) 95-107.

26.   I.K. Ashton, V. Sahota, D. Lindsay and B.A. Ashton, *Calcif. Tiss. Internat.* **52** (1993) S12.

27.   J.L. Henry, *Agents and Actions* **41** (1993) 75-87.

CHAPTER 10

GROWTH AND DEVELOPMENT OF THE
LUMBAR VERTEBRAL CANAL

R.W. Porter

1. The importance of the lumbar vertebral canal

The vertebral canal is the anatomical space bounded by the vertebrae and discs anteriorly, the pedicles laterally and the neural arch posteriorly. The ligamentum flavum is the immediate posterior soft tissue relation in the intervertebral space, with the posterior longitudinal ligament anteriorly. Within the canal, the cauda equina in its envelope of dura, and the exiting nerve roots at each segmental level, are separated from the canal boundaries, Batson's plexus of veins, and extradural fat.

The dura occupies approximately 66% of the space within the vertebral canal, leaving adequate room for encroaching pathology, without any neurological compromise. Neither disc protrusion nor osteophytes affect the neurological structures when the canal is of reasonable size. However archaeological studies show that there is a great variation in size and shape of the vertebral canal, and in a few individuals the dura is tightly packed and there is little extradural space to accommodate pathology.

We first used ultrasound to measure the 15 degree oblique diameter of the lumbar vertebral canal two decades ago[1], reporting that approximately 50% of patients admitted with symptomatic lumbar disc protrusion, had canals in the bottom ten percent of the asymptomatic population. We concluded that patients with wider canals presumably had disc pathology, but that the presence of symptoms depended on the canal size (Figures 1 and 2). Similarly we observed that in patients with root entrapment syndrome from degenerative change and in patients with neurogenic claudication, the vertebral canal tended to be narrow[2]. These results have been supported by subsequent studies using CT and MRI, demonstrating that the size of the vertebral canal is an important factor in the multifactorial aetiology of cauda equina and root lesions.

It might be argued that individuals with a small vertebral canal have small neural contents and are therefore not disadvantaged. At times this may be true, but clinical experience shows that there are many patients with neurological spine disorders who have the dura is packed tightly within a small trefoil canal. A possible mechanism is explained below.

2. The growth of the vertebral canal

We examined 155 juvenile and 836 adult archaeological vertebrae from Romano British and Anglo-Saxon collections. We observed that the vertebral canal of small children was of adult size by four years of age (Figure 3). Infants had a cross sectional area and mid-sagittal diameter equivalent to adult size. The interpedicular diameter however continued to grow up to puberty[3] (Figure 4).

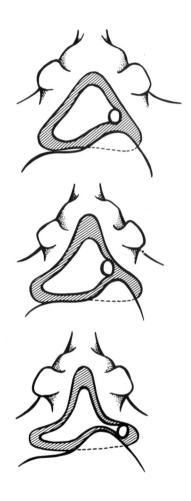

Figure 1. A diagram showing a triangular shaped canal above, a more trefoil shaped canal in the centre, and a markedly trefoil canal below. A disc protrusion of similar size may spare the nerve root in a large canal, but compromise the root when space is limited.

All the long bones of the skeleton were compared with the canal parameters, and there was no single useful correlation between the mid-sagittal diameter and other bones. However there was a relationship between the mid-sagittal diameter and the combined length of the clavicle, the skull circumference and discrepancy in leg length. It is of

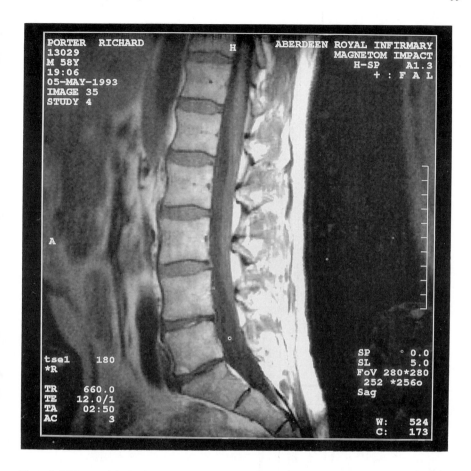

Figure 2. MRI scan of the lumbar spine. The L4/5 disc is compatible with disc degeneration and a posterior disc bulge. The vertebral canal is wide, perhaps explaining occasional back pain, but no root symptoms.

interest that the clavicle is the first bone to ossify, and that leg length inequality may be related to subtle impairment of foetal development, and the skull adapts to the size of its contents.

The interpedicular diameter correlated well with the width of the vertebral body, and with the length of the femur. Thus tall individuals tended to have large vertebrae and wide pedicles, but stature was unrelated to the mid-sagittal diameter and area.

Further archaeological studies examining 700 skeletons from the Spittalfield collection at the Natural History Museum (where the exact date of death is known), has shown that the area and mid sagittal diameter is mature at one year of age at L1-L4, and at L5 by four years of age[4].

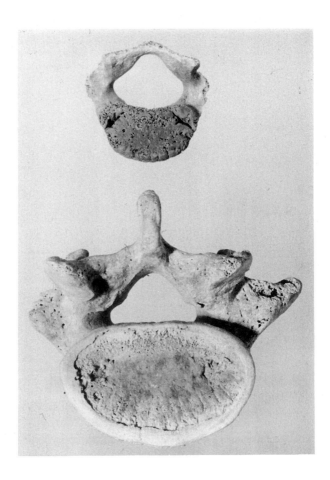

Figure 3. The fifth lumbar vertebra of a four year old child compared with an adult in the same Romano British population. The area and the mid sagittal diameters are the same.

3. Environmental factors

George Clark suggested that infant malnutrition may significantly impair the growth of the vertebral canal at a critical time[5], and that the canal may not have further growth potential. There may be environmental factors which stunt the growing canal, and in the absence of catch-up growth, that canal remains small throughout life. We examined the canal size in three archaeological populations and observed a positive correlation with

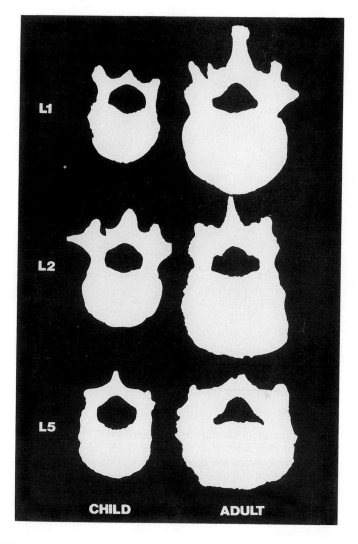

Figure 4. Silhouette photographs of representative vertebrae at L1, L2 and L5 in an infant and in an adult from an Anglo Saxon population. The mid sagittal diameters are the same, but the interpedicular diameters are greater in the adult.

physiological stress indicators[6]. Thus it is probable that adverse conditions *in-utero* affect the neuro-osseous development, and leave the fossil of spinal stenosis.

If other sensitive growing systems were similarly affected, we would expect to find that patients with spinal stenosis were disadvantaged. In a number of studies we have

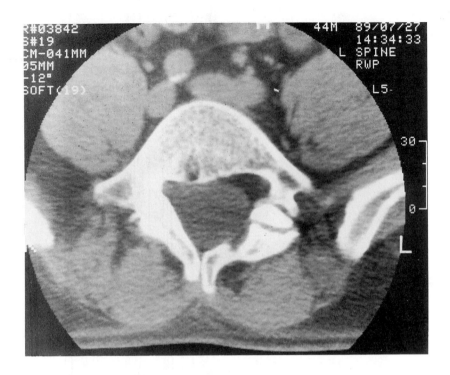

Figure 5. CT scan of a patient with spina bifida and unilateral spondylolysis, showing a wide canal.

noted reduced intellectual ability in subjects with small canals. In a group of 16 year old school children, those with smaller canals compared less favourably than those with larger canals[7] though their stature was similar. In a health assessment, patients with wider canals had more post school qualifications than those with smaller canals[8]. These same subjects with wider canals had significantly less cardiovascular and digestive problems than those with narrower canals. It is probable that during a window of opportunity, environmental factors adversely affect not only the growing spine, but also the neurological and immune systems.

4. The trefoil canal

This concept provides a hypothesis for the development of the small trefoil shaped vertebral canal. At L5 the vertebral canal is trefoil in shape in about 15% of the population. We have noted that there is a correlation between the trefoil shape and a small mid-sagittal diameter, an unhealthy combination if that canal is compromised by

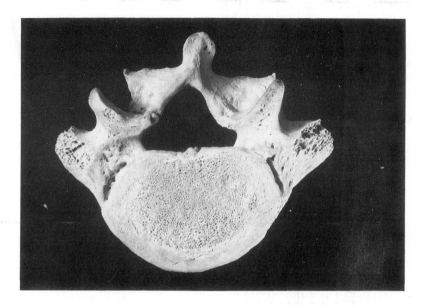

Figure 6. A fifth lumbar vertebra with a unilateral spondylolysis, showing a large vertebral canal.

pathology. The dural sac and its contents then have little reserve capacity. We suggest that during intra uterine life, there is an environmental insult to growth which affects the spinal cord and the surrounding bony canal. In the foetus when the spinal cord is in the sacrum, the vertebral canal probably adapts to the size of its contents, much as the skull epigenetically conforms to the size of the brain. Then in the last trimester, as the small cord rises in the small canal, the canal probably still matches its contents. The baby grows with an improved environment, developing a large stature, wide vertebrae and wide pedicles. The large long bones are matched by large muscles and a large cauda equina. However, the area and mid sagittal diameter of the lumbar spine remain small. As the child reaches maturity, the pedicles widen out, but with a small mid sagittal diameter, the canal the becomes trefoil in shape.

5. Spina bifida and spondylolysis

There are two developmental pathologies which are a bonus for the vertebral canal. The first is spina bifida occulta. For long this was thought to be a innocuous condition. Our studies suggest that as regards the canal, spina bifida occulta confers an advantage. The segment proximal to the lesion is wider than the mean size for the rest of the population[9], reducing the risk of neural compromise (Figure 5). Surgeons rarely encounter a bifid neural arch when operating on a disc protrusion, not because protrusions are uncommon in these patients, but because the extra space confers a margin of safety for the nerve roots.

Secondly, in the presence of spondylolysis the area and mid sagittal diameters are relatively large, again protecting these patients from neurological symptoms at the more proximal level. Unilateral spondylolysis is similarly associated with a wide canal[10] (Figure 6).

6. Conclusion

Spinal stenosis and the neurological compromise in patients with disc protrusion, root entrapment and claudication, is responsible for a large component of lumbar spine disability. A search for factors which in early life affect the canal's growth could be rewarding, with considerable medical, social and economic significance.

7. References

1. R.W. Porter, M. Wicks, C. Hibbert, *J. Bone Joint Surg.* **60-B** (1978) 485-487.
2. R.W. Porter, C. Hibbert, F. Wellman, *Spine* **8** (1980) 99-105.
3. R.W. Porter, *Thesis*, University of Edinburgh (1980).
4. T. Papp, R.W. Porter, *Spine* (in press).
5. G.A. Clark, M.M. Panjabi, F.T. Wetzel, *Spine* **10** (1985) 165-170.
6. R.W. Porter, D. Pavitt, *Spine* **12** (1987) 901-906.
7. R.W. Porter, J.N. Drinkall, D.E. Porter, L. Thorp, *Spine* **12** (1987) 907-911.
8. R.W. Porter, G. Oakshott, *Spine* **19** (1994) 901-903.
9. T. Papp, R.W. Porter, *Spine* **19** (1994) 1508-1511.
10. R.W. Porter, W. Park, *J. Bone Joint Surg.* **45-B** (1982) 39-59.

CHAPTER 11

PATHOLOGICAL CHANGES CONTRIBUTING TO BACK PAIN AND SCIATICA

J.A.N. Shepperd

1. Introduction

This chapter aims to address patterns of degenerative change seen in cadave specimens, and thereby speculate on painful as opposed to painless situations.

Ageing changes are invariably seen in the lumbar spine and quite commonly may be present by the third decade of life. Such changes may be associated with pain, but the relationship is often obscure. Contrary to popular belief, physical excesses and manual work seem frequently to be associated with relatively little back pain disability (compared with sedentary workers). X-ray evidence is considered highly unreliable as a predictor of back pain (ref). Furthermore in an age which sees increasingly less physical work and shorter working hours, the remorseless rise of working hours lost through back pain suggests that degenerative change *per se* may have little relevance. Following from the clinical experience of provocative testing (ref.) it seems probable that a major source of pain in the back is the highly innervated posterior longitudinal ligament along where it is attached to the intervertebral disc (ref.)(Table 1). Coupled with irritation of the outer theca and perhaps pressure on sensitive nerves within the end plate, it seems likely that the majority of pain in the back has its source from this specific anatomical region. Possible inflammatory agents include mechanical factors such as disc protrusion, abnormal compression or distraction of the posterior disc, and hydrostatic influences whereby intradiscal fluid is forced under high pressure through deficient structures. Chemical factors are also considered possible causative agents such as findings of raised levels of neuropeptides in the vicinity of a spondylitic back (ref.), leukotrines (ref.) and other possible inflammatory agents. In addition autoimmune aspects have been suggested (ref).

This same list probably applies equally to nerve root dysfunction and pain, but in addition the root is probably affected by interference with circulation (ref.) either in the form of scarring or in association with a systemic disease such as diabetes.

Table 1. Breakdown of diagnoses produced from probing of 321 spinal segments in 154 patients

Diagnosis	No. of patients
Facet joint alone	29
Disc annulus alone	53
Facet and disc	45
Diffuse pain, no firm diagnosis	27

2. Biomechanics of the nucleus pulposus

In order to assess these aspects, cadaver studies were undertaken in which fresh post mortem specimens were retrieved as sagittal divided half spines from L3 to the sacrum. The initial study included 100 specimens with a sampling from all ages of life from neonate through to old age (Table 2). The specimens were deep frozen and then surfaced by planing with a sharp blade to produce a clean surface (Figure 1). The specimens were mounted in a frame and subjected to compression and distraction. Following this, loaded flexion and extension were studied, recorded by x-ray, photography and video.

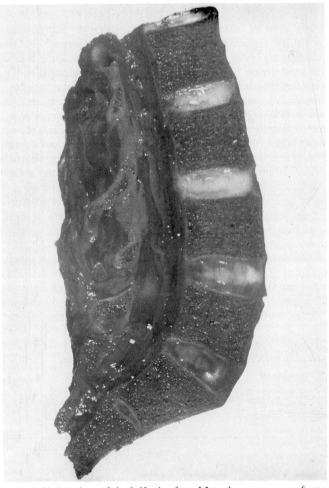

Figure 1. Sagitally divided sections of the half-spine from L3 to the sacrum were frozen, planed and mounted.

Table 2. 100 Sagittal cadaver half spines

Age	Specimens	Discs
0-10	3	7
10-20	2	5
20-30	8	16
30-40	6	12
40-50	13	23
50-60	15	35
60-70	17	31
70-80	19	42
80+	17	40
	100	223

In early life the nucleus and inner annulus are tethered by collagen fibres to end plate cartilage and bone (Figure 2). End plate pressure is borne by the annulus and nucleus in varying ratios depending on the hydration of the nucleus. The hydrostatic pressure of the nucleus is maintained by trapped proteoglycans within the collagen matrix of its own structure, and acts like a sponge. It is therefore, not normally liable to explode or extrude and the act of nucleotomy has little effect on a normal young disc. The whole structure from annulus to end plate nucleus appears integrated by between adolescence and early adult life, a clear boundary develops between the nucleus and end plate cartilage which represents a fault line. This boundary is readily demonstrated by discography, but distraction of such a disc fails to reveal an obvious fissure. By mid-thirties however, the fault line has become a fissure with an obvious cavity demonstrable on distraction. This fissure passes both further anterior and posterior and in a coronal section extends laterally. Such changes are more prevalent in the lower two discs than L3 but were found at least in one level in every specimen from the mid-forties. In older specimens, extension of these fissures occurs initially posterior and sometimes anterior with a vertebral fissure usually reflecting distally. In coronal section, these fissures extend laterally often into a 'bag' at the edge of the disc. This lateral 'bag' may be seen as a syndesmophyte extending laterally on x-ray although the obliquity of the usual AP view, which is centred on the mid-lumbar spine, generally obscures this feature.

These degenerative cavities within a disc have been referred to as a vacuum effect (ref.) although this idea is probably a misrepresentation. The space which can be generated on distraction would cause negative pressure and changing from the standing to the lying position would also generate temporary negative pressure although conversely changing from the lying to the standing position, would generate positive pressure. The space will inevitably in time fill with mainly nitrogen gas and occasionally such gas can be demonstrated expelled into the epidural space (Figure 3). The pattern seen in cadaver specimens are equally well demonstrated by discography.

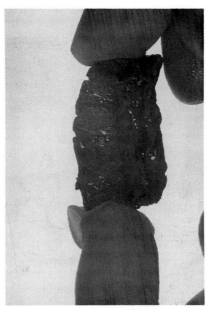

Figure 2. A neonatal specimen in which the nucleus and annulus are less distinct. By early adult life a fault line arises generating a 'hamburger' discogram. By mid-life the fault lines develop into fissures anteriorly, posteriorly and in the coronal plane.

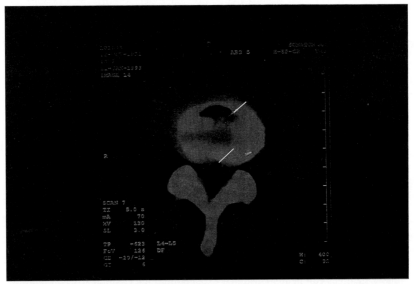

Figure 3. CT scan showing intradiscal gas within a fissure, some of which has been expelled through the defective annulus into the spinal canal and is resting anterior to the theca.

3. Effects of movement

Movement of the spine produces characteristic dynamics of the nucleus. In flexion the nucleus moves posteriorly and in extension it moves anteriorly (Figure 4). This consistent feature means that the motion segment joint is polycentric. The range of movement varied among the individual specimens examined regardless of age. The material of individual disc specimens is significantly varied.

Movement is greater when the nucleus is more hydrated. Hydration is achieved in the *in vitro* specimen by exposing it to a saline swab. Because of the forward and backward movement, shear forces occur at the fixed end plate boundary and the mobile nucleus boundary and coincide with the fault line referred to above, which is seen between adolescence and early adult life. This horizontal H configuration seen on discography is often referred to as the normal 'hamburger' discogram. It is well known that the collagen component of the nucleus increases with age, possibly as a repair attempt from the continual shearing forces which arise within its structure. Changes gradually extend towards the disc periphery.

Buckling and disruption of the inner posterior annulus are commonly seen by the mid-thirties which tie in with the grinding rotation movement seen within the annulus on anterior and posterior flexion. Coronal cut sections reveal corresponding changes in the lateral plane, which correspond with the movements of bipedal gait, thus flexion to the right causes shift of nuclear material to the left, and flexion to the left causes nuclear material to move to the right. This development of cavities and portals within the intervertebral disc in conjunction with loose material particularly that of the inner posterior annulus, sets the scene for patterns of disc herniation. It is well known that disc herniation on the one hand is highly prevalent and also that its correlation with symptom production is at times vague (ref.). The influence of herniation is both the production of physical pressure on nerves and also the provocation of inflammatory change. When a hernia becomes established the typical pattern is one of exacerbation and remission of symptoms, although repeat scans of the hernia will usually show little obvious change.

Patterns of late disc disruption include extension of the fault line into a vertical anterior fissure which mirrors the line of the facet joint and corresponds to a profound lowering of the centre of movement of the motion segment from a point in the upper part of the lower vertebral body, to a region several centimetres lower. This altered axis of movement will certainly contribute to disruptive shearing at the facet joint and may contribute to degenerative spondylolisthesis. Post mortem specimens nevertheless indicate this type of situation where it is highly mobile, and also where it is apparently fused and stabilised representing an event earlier in the individual's life. In this situation, inflammatory change from the facet joint would be capable of involving the nerve root in the lateral recess.

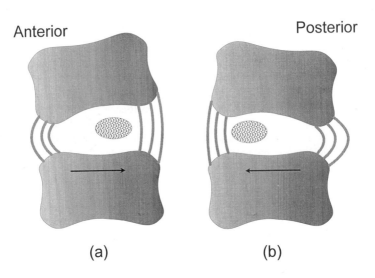

Figure 4. In flexion the nucleus moves posteriorly and in extension it moves anteriorly.

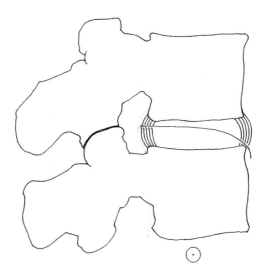

Figure 5. Late disruption of the disc frequently produces an anterior vertical fissure mirroring the line of the facet joint. This lowers the centre of motion and damages the facet joint.

4. Muscles and ligaments

The significance of muscle control and ligament control in degenerative disc development could be the key to the surprising fact that the sedentary worker appears more vulnerable to symptomatology than the manual worker. A model was produced in which dynamic and static posterior muscle control was represented by a fixed polyester and an elastic band held on a lever. A fixed turning moment was applied on the upper end plate. With no muscle substitution at all, the amount of angular displacement for a fixed turning moment was predictably the greatest and consequently the displacement of intradiscal material was also the greatest (Figure 6). The presence of posterior dynamic muscle is to reduce the amount of angular displacement whilst the intradiscal compression remains constant. Or conversely, to achieve the same amount of angular displacement in the amuscular condition requires a greater turning force and thereby greater compression on the disc. It is possible that low pressure displacement of the disc causes more shearing than high pressure displacement of the intradiscal material. The presence of a fixed check-rein limits the displacement of intradiscal material and angular displacement regardless of turning moment. Sudden release of the fixed posterior control, such as will happen with reflex inhibition of the erector spinae, will generate a highly destructive shock wave throughout the posterior disc. The combination of a painful experience and resulting muscle inhibition such as may occur bending over to tie up a shoe lace, is likely in combination to cause disruption of the disc.

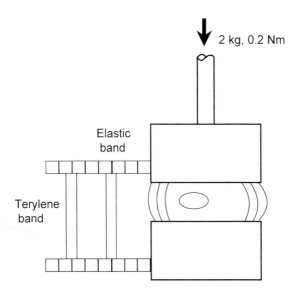

Figure 6. Diagram of model with specimen mounted to represent dynamic and static muscle control.

5. Centre of movement, resultant force and intradiscal displacement

Centre of movement can be analysed by studying sequential frozen images on a video. Whilst variations occur, in a normal disc, the centre of movement is invariably polycentric. In the neutral position it lies in the upper third of the vertebral body below (Figure 7), with forward flexion it moves forward, ending, at its extreme, just anterior to the lower end plate. In extension it moves backwards ending, at its furthest extent, within the posterior longitudinal ligament at disc level. Where patterns of derangement have occurred the centre of movement also varies (Figure 8).

The resultant applied load likewise moves anteriorly in flexion and posteriorly in extension. The loading across the normal disc is believed to range between 1000 and 1500 N (ref.). Whilst the fluid-like structure of nucleus achieves uniform hydrostatic pressure, the annulus is a visco-elastic solid and behaves in a different way. Flexion increases compression in the anterior nucleus and distraction in the posterior nucleus, while extension achieves the opposite. When the nucleus is under-hydrated the annulus bears an increasing proportion of the load and estimates from bone density studies have suggested that the normal ratio is approximately twice as much load on the annulus as the nucleus.

Detailed analysis of annular material on the video indicates that the posterior annulus undergoes a rotary movement within its substance. This rotation is approximately three times the angular movement of the segment. The anterior annulus on the other hand, appears to undergo within its substance, a shearing displacement angled approximately 45 degrees caudad. When the anterior annulus undergoes failure this shearing force is represented by a caudally reflected anterior vertical fissure.

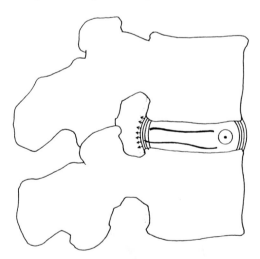

Figure 7. The centre of motion in the sagittal plane varies according to the positions of the vertebrae. In the neutral position it lies in the upper third of the lower vertebral body.

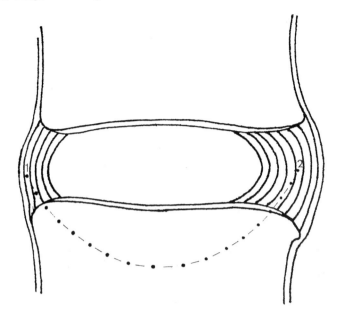

Figure 8. A complete front-to-back fissure lowers the centre of movement and a simple posterior fissure moves the axis anteriorly.

In these circumstances the centre of rotation is profoundly affected and becomes far lower in the vertebral body below the motion segment.

The fact that the bulk movement of the intradiscal material is in the opposite direction to the centre of load underscores the shearing forces which exist within the disc.

6. Conclusion

By studying the motion of a sagitally divided section, it is possible to observe the internal structure of the disc. Whilst interference with the disc may be thought to affect the validity of the observations, the findings are so consistent that we believe they provide an important insight into the mechanism of disc degeneration. The potentially harmful distortion of the disc structure would certainly be increased by weak muscle control and it is possible that this is a contributing factor to the increasing incidence of back disability in the late 20th Century.

7. References

1.   J.A.N. Shepperd, in *Management of Back Pain*, 2nd ed., R.W. Porter
        (Churchill-Livingstone, 1993) pp. 161-163.
2.   K. Olmarker, J. Blomquist, J. Strömberg, U. Nannmark, P. Thomsen and
        B. Rydevik, *Trans. ISSLS*, 1993, Seattle, p.12.
3.   S.D. Boden, D.O. Davis, T.S. Dina, N.J. Patronas and S.W. Wiesel *J.
        Bone Joint Surg.* **72-A** (1990) 403.
4.   R.M. Aspden, *Spine* **14** (1989) 266.

CHAPTER 12

MEASUREMENT OF VERTEBRAL BLOOD FLOW AND ITS SIGNIFICANCE IN DISC DISEASE

A.M.C. Thomas, G.F. Keenan and M. Brown

1. Introduction

Bone and soft tissue blood flow are of importance in bone growth, fracture healing and many metabolic and structural disorders of bone in man. Disturbances of blood flow may produce pathological changes in both the adult and in the growing child for example Perthes disease, Keinbocks disease and avascular necrosis of the hip.

The intervertebral disc depends on diffusion of oxygen and nutrients from surrounding structures. The principle routes of diffusion are through the vertebral end plate and through the periphery of the annulus of the intervertebral disc[1]. Disturbances in vertebral end plate blood flow may obviously impair the nutrition of the intervertebral disc and may result in premature intervertebral disc degeneration. This may explain the relatively higher incidence of premature intervertebral disc degeneration in smokers[2]. The passage of nutrients from the end plate circulation to the disc may depend on mechanical factors such as cycles of loading and unloading[3] and this may explain differences in intervertebral disc degeneration in office workers and ambulant workers. Disturbances in blood supply may also result from mechanical vibration. The circulation within the intervertebral body and in the subchondral bone of the vertebral end plate has been described by Crock[4]. A study of those disorders caused by abnormal blood flow requires a reliable method by which to quantify changes in blood flow. Bone blood flow has been notoriously difficult to measure quantitatively and accurately. Since bony organs do not have a discrete vascular hilum supplying and draining them, the application of the Fick principle to measure blood flow is therefore not entirely reliable.

The gold standard for experimental measurement of bone blood flow is the microsphere technique[5]. Many studies of various sites in animals have been performed using this technique. However it is invasive in nature and unsuitable for studies in man. A technique for *in vivo* measurement of regional blood flow in man has been developed in Aberdeen[6]. Using ^{15}O-labelled water and Positron Emission Tomography (PET) we can quantify bone and soft tissue blood flow in man. Initial work has been done on blood flow at the site of a tibial fracture. Recently attention has turned to vertebral body perfusion.

At present studies have been conducted to establish base line normal values for vertebral body blood flow using the microsphere reference organ method in an animal model and positron emission tomography in the human adult.

2. Microsphere studies

2.1. Method

In the microsphere method 15 μm diameter polystyrene microspheres are used. The microspheres are radio-labelled with [85]Strontium. A known number of microspheres are injected into the left ventricle of the animal to be studied using a catheter. The microspheres distribute themselves around the body and are trapped in capillaries. The diameter of sphere is chosen to ensure a high percentage of entrapment without using an excessively large sphere. The lungs are routinely counted at the end of the experiment to check the percentage of entrapment. The microspheres are assumed to distribute themselves around the body to each organ and the number trapped in that organ therefore depends on the proportion of the cardiac output going to that organ. At the same time as the injection is given a catheter is placed in a large artery and blood is withdrawn from it at a known rate. The activity in the sample is therefore the activity expected in an organ with the same blood flow as the syringe. At the conclusion of the experiment the animal is killed and the spine is removed and dissected. It is not necessary to kill the animal immediately after the microsphere injection as the microspheres are assumed to remain entrapped in the capillaries and it is therefore possible using different isotopes to make repeated blood flow measurements. During dissection of the spine great care is required to remove all the surrounding soft tissue from the vertebrae as one of the major potential problems with this technique is contamination of bone samples with muscle. Muscle has higher blood flow than bone and therefore contains more microspheres. The laminae, pedicles and facet joints were therefore not included in the samples but the cartilaginous end plates were left *in situ*. The blood flow measurements were carried out in a single 20 kg dog and four mature New Zealand red rabbits and expressed as a fraction of the body weight.

2.2. Results

Dissection of the vertebral bodies in both species showed a progressive increase in size in the caudal direction. There was only a very thin cortex in all vertebral bodies. This is important as cortical bone has a relatively lower blood flow than cancellous bone and would thus reduce the average blood flow. In the dog model we studied the measurements showed a range of vertebral flow rates from 12.7 ml/min/100 g at the T9 level to 6.5 ml/min/100 g at the L5 level. The flow rates in the lumbar vertebral bodies were significantly lower than in the thoracic region. There were calculated to be several hundred microspheres in each bone sample in the dog and we therefore have a high degree of confidence that the flow rates measured in this particular animal are accurate. In the rabbits the dissection is much more difficult and the bone samples are much smaller. This means that the samples contain fewer microspheres and thus the flow rates obtainable tend to be less accurate. We found that typical values ranged from 10 to 25 ml/min/100 g. A tendency to lower flows in the lumbar region was seen in one animal. This effect was not so marked as in the dog and in the other rabbits the flow was similar throughout the spines within the limits of error of the technique; 21 ± 3 ml/min/100 g at T8, 18 ± 3 at L1 and 16 ± 3 at L5.

3. Sickle-cell disease

In clinical practice there are conditions in which structures of similar size to microspheres are present in the circulation and potentially embolised to the vertebrae. An example of this is in disseminated tuberculosis. The distribution of spinal tuberculosis has long been recognised to follow a clear pattern with the maximum incidence occurring in the thoracolumbar junction region. This maximal incidence is different to the maximal incidence of symptomatic intervertebral disc degeneration which is highest in the low lumbar region. In sickle-cell anaemia abnormally shaped red cells result in clumping and there are alterations in blood viscosity. This produces disturbances of circulation and infarction of various organs in the skeleton, the most important areas clinically are the femoral head and humeral head. In the spine sickle-cell anaemia produces a characteristic picture of scalloping of the vertebral end plate. Older papers on this subject have suggested that repeated vertebral infarction leads to crush fractures in the vertebral bodies. This process however will be expected to occur in a random fashion as in osteoporotic crush fractures. The damage in sickle-cell anaemia is much more uniform and is present in younger patients. A review of the literature revealed no systematic study of this phenomena and we therefore reviewed the records of 100 patients attending sickle-cell anaemia clinics in three centres. We found 20 patients who had, at some time, complained of low back pain sufficiently severe to warrant a spinal x-ray. We reviewed these lumbar spine films and ten sets of films exhibited the typical sickle-cell changes and 10 sets of films did not. (Obviously we don't know the incidence of the abnormality in the 80 patients who were asymptomatic). The vertebral bodies were analysed by measuring the height of the front and back of the vertebral body on the lateral whole lumbar spine radiograph, measuring the height of the vertebral body where it was maximally depressed and calculating a percentage end plate depression. The condition showed a clear pattern with the damage being more severe in the thoracolumbar junction region in the affected patients. The distribution of the abnormality appeared to be similar to the levels effected in spinal tuberculosis.

In view of the potential effect of the blood flow changes on intervertebral disc nutrition and in an attempt to establish the incidence of the changes in asymptomatic patients we approached all patients attending the sickle-cell anaemia clinic in Birmingham and asked them to attend for an MRI scan of the lumbar spine. We also asked other patients attending the Royal Orthopaedic Hospital with sickle-cell anaemia to have a lumbar MRI scan. Unfortunately it proved difficult to recruit many patients but 8 patients did have lumbar MRI for the purposes of this study. The MRI scans revealed that the vertebral body changes are present in young patients, the youngest being aged 20. However the vertebral body changes, even when severe, did not necessarily result in premature intervertebral disc degeneration.

4. Positron emission tomography

Accurate measurement of regional blood flow *in vivo* in man is difficult. Over the last three years a method of quantifying blood flow in man has been developed using positron emission tomography. Initial studies of blood flow in fracture healing have shown the method to be accurate and reproducible.

We have made estimates of vertebral body blood flow using this technique. This is more complex than measurement of tibial blood flow as it involves a preliminary MRI scan which is then warped onto the PET scan to define regions of interest. Values obtained for perfusion in lumbar vertebral bodies using PET are comparable to those obtained in microsphere studies.

4.1. Method

The patient has an MRI examination taking images transaxially through the chosen vertebral body. Oil filled tubes placed on the skin are seen as high intensity signals on the images. These tubes are then replaced by germanium sources during the PET studies. Having these locating devices around the scans allows subsequent warping, or overlaying, of the PET and MRI images on each other for the purposes of analysis. Arterial and venous cannulae are each inserted under local anaesthetic into radial artery at the wrist and a suitable vein on the contralateral hand.

^{15}O labelled water is prepared by bombarding nitrogen with 15 MeV deuterons from the Aberdeen CS-30 cyclotron using the ^{14}N (d,n) ^{15}O reaction. The resulting ^{15}O-labelled oxygen is then combined with hydrogen using a palladium catalyst.

Tomography is performed using an EG and G Ortec ECAT II tomograph (CTI West Inc, California, USA). To obtain images at each level, approximately 1850 MBq of ^{15}O-labelled water, in about 4 ml of saline, were injected into the arm through an intravenous cannula. Continuous arterial blood sampling, monitored using a beta counter, gives decay data to produce an activity time course curve, allowing absolute quantification of blood flow. The attenuation corrected images were analysed using software developed in house (PET SHOP, C.Goddard) on a SUN SPARC work station.

4.2. Results

Mean count values are obtained using region of interest (ROI) technique over the vertebra. Using arterial decay information the absolute flow values may be calculated.

Using this method we have obtained perfusion figures similar to that measured by microspheres in animals: an average of 7.6 ml/min/100 g with a range of 4.2 to 10.8 ml/min/100 g.

5. Discussion

The experiments presented have established that there is probably a regional variation in vertebral body blood flow both in our animal model, and in human subjects. The clinical correlates of this variation are seen in spinal tuberculosis and sickle-cell anaemia. It would be interesting to know whether the changes in sickle-cell anaemia are present in younger patients prior to ossification of the vertebral end plate epiphysis. Although the changes observed do not necessarily result in premature intervertebral disc degeneration nevertheless it would be interesting to know whether the observed changes do tend to result in premature disc degeneration in older adults. This information may help in studies of the intractable problem of chronic severe low back pain in sickle-cell anaemia patients.

We are at present evaluating a high resolution multisection PET scanner and we will be using this technique to examine vertebral blood flow changes following exercise in patients with neurogenic claudication. The study of vertebral body blood flow using microsphere and PET techniques will undoubtedly bring new understanding to the pathophysiology and natural history of many conditions of the spine.

6. Acknowledgements

We thank the Arthritis and Rheumatism Council, the ROH Orthopaedic Trust, the Wishbone Foundation and the Welcome Trust for financial support. We are especially grateful to the Haematologists and Radiologists at the London Hospital, Newham District Hospital, Queen Elizabeth Hospital, Birmingham and the Royal Orthopaedic Hospital for their help with execution of some of these studies.

7. References

1.   K. Ogatat and L.A. Whiteside, *Clin. Orthop.* **170** (1982) 296.

2.   T. Battie and K. Gill, *Spine* **16** (1991) 1015.

3.   J.P.G. Urban, S. Holm, A. Maroudas and A. Nachemson, *Clin. Orthop.* **170** (1982) 296.

4.   H.V. Crock, M. Goldwasser and H. Yoshizawa, In *The Biology of the Intervertebral Disc*, ed P. Ghosh (CRC Press, Florida, 1989) p.109.

5.   G. Li, J.T. Bronk and P.J. Kelly, *J. Orthop. Res.* **7** (1989) 61.

6.   G.P. Ashcroft, R.W. Porter, N.T.S Evans, D. Roeda, C. Goddard and F.W. Smith, *J. Bone Joint Surg.* **74-B** (1992) 324.

8.   G.P. Ashcroft, N.T.S. Evans, D. Roeda, M. Dodd, J.R. Mallard, R.W. Porter and F.W. Smith, *J. Bone Joint Surg.* **74-B:** (1992) 673.

CHAPTER 13

THE PATHOPHYSIOLOGY OF NEUROGENIC CLAUDICATION

R.W. Porter

1. Definitions

The term "claudication of the spinal cord" was first used by DeJerine[1] when describing patients with claudication symptoms who had normal peripheral pulses. Van Gelderen[2] reported a patient with root symptoms which appeared on walking, but which were relieved by rest. He thought this was due to thickening of the ligamentum flavum. Bermark[3] described "intermittent spinal claudication" attributing a neurospinal origin to the walking pains of two patients. However it was Verbiest in 1954[4] who recognised that structural narrowing of the vertebral canal could compress the cauda equina producing claudication symptoms. The clinical presentation is now better defined, and we know that the pathology is multifactorial in origin.

'Neurogenic claudication' is a term which should be reserved for the patient with spinal stenosis, whilst 'intermittent claudication' is associated with peripheral vascular disease. It is sometimes overdiagnosed. Many patients have pains in their legs when walking, or pains aggravated by walking, which are sometimes loosely called claudication pain, but such a description is inaccurate unless the symptoms are clearly defined. Neurogenic claudication is not present at rest, but it affects one or both legs after the patient has been walking a short distance. They experience pain or discomfort, tiredness or heaviness, which increases as they walk, and they have to stop. The symptoms settle down and they can walk again. By definition such patients must have a degree of spinal stenosis to warrant the diagnosis.

2. Differential diagnosis

Peripheral vascular disease often coexists with neurogenic claudication[5]. Posture can dramatically affect the walking distance in neurogenic claudication and discriminate from intermittent claudication[6] (Figure 1). Back pain which is referred to the thighs at rest and which is aggravated by walking is not claudication. Patients with root entrapment pain associated with degenerative changes in the root canal, may experience an increase in their pain as they walk, but again this is not claudication. Walking pain can be an inappropriate symptom in patients with abnormal pain behaviour, and if there are many inappropriate signs, the diagnosis should be reconsidered. Other causes of walking pain need to be excluded, such as degenerative change of the hip, venous insufficiency, and myxoedema.

3. Developmental stenosis

Patients with neurogenic claudication generally have a developmentally narrow canal

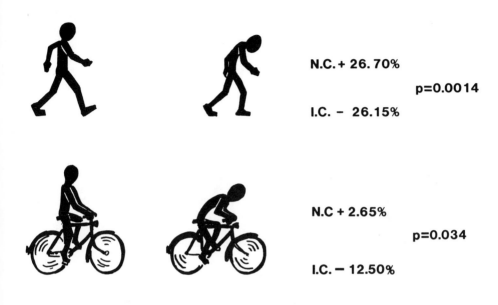

N.C. + 26. 70%

p=0.0014

I.C. - 26.15%

N.C + 2.65%

p=0.034

I.C. - 12.50%

Figure 1. The median percentage differences in walking and cycling tolerance by flexing forward in 19 patients with neurogenic claudication and 11 with intermittent claudication. As a population stooping forwards increased the distances in neurogenic claudication, but for individual patients this is not a good discriminator.

throughout the spine. They have had a small canal from childhood, but only recently developed symptoms. Occasionally the patient has a stenotic achondroplastic spine. Many patients with stenotic canals never have claudication pain. MRI studies of asymptomatic subjects over 60 years of age show spinal stenosis in 21%[7]. The canal is therefore but one factor in the pathology.

4. Degenerative stenosis

A second factor is the degenerative change associated with heavy manual work. Few patients have been sedentary workers. The high male incidence may be related to the heavier manual work. Thickening of the ligamentum flavum[8] or ossification[9] may be responsible for the stenosis, usually at the inter segmental level. Diffuse idiopathic spinal hyperostosis (DISH) can precipitate stenosis, when this is associated with a developmentally small canal.

5. Vertebral displacement

If the canal is already narrow, segmental displacement in the sagittal plane, or rotatory displacement can cause a critical problem. Degenerative spondylolisthesis effectively reduces the canal size at the level of displacement. Although degenerative spondylolisthesis is more common in women than in men, half of the men with neurogenic claudication in our series have degenerative spondylolisthesis[10]. Women with this displacement infrequently develop claudication. However many patients with unilateral claudication and lumbar scoliosis are women.

6. Abnormal nerve function

The neuropathology of claudication is probably the result of inadequate oxygenation, or accumulation of metabolites in the cauda equina. Nerve function is just adequate at rest, but not during exercise. The effect of compression on nerve function has been extensively studied in animal experiments[11-13], but how this is related to chronic stenosis and walking is speculative.

7. Central stenosis at one level does not explain claudication

Although it is not possible to make a diagnosis of neurogenic claudication without central canal stenosis, there are a number of clinical reasons why central stenosis alone will not explain the mechanism. First a slowly growing spinal tumour can occlude the canal, but not cause claudication (Figure 2). Secondly, a massive disc protrusion can block the canal, and not cause claudication (Figure 3). Thirdly a single level stenosis not uncommonly occludes the flow in a radiculogram, but may not cause claudication. Furthermore, imaging of asymptomatic subjects shows that many have stenosis, and claudicating patients have had stenosis for many years before their first symptoms. Again it is surprising that in canine studies, a 25% constriction of the cauda equina may not cause a neurological deficit.

8. Root canal stenosis does not explain the symptoms of claudication

A number of authors have thought that root canal stenosis or foraminal stenosis is responsible for claudication[14-17]. However isolated stenosis of the root canal can be asymptomatic, and when it is associated with symptoms, it is generally constant root pain even at rest. If the root canal is important, why do claudicating patients invariably have central stenosis?

9. Two level low pressure stenosis - venous congestion

Imaging studies of patients with neurogenic claudication show that many have multiple levels of stenosis. We have examined 50 patients with neurogenic claudication using radiculography and CT, and 47 of them had multiple levels of stenosis, either in the central canal, or in the central canal at one level and the root canal distally,[10]

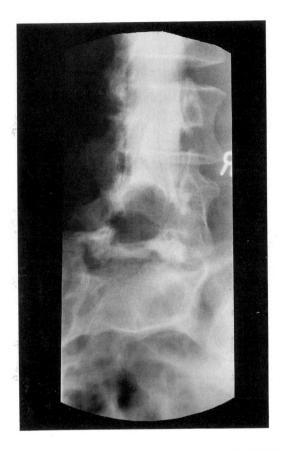

Figure 2. A radiculogram in a patient with chronic back pain and a spondylolisthesis. They also had large paraganglionoma occluding the canal. There were no claudication symptoms.

(Figure 4). Two of the three with a single level of central stenosis, had a lumbar scoliosis and unilateral claudication (Figure 5). The third had marked peripheral vascular disease. Clinically multiple levels of stenosis seems to be significant.

A two level concept agrees with previously reported clinical observations[18]. McGuire and colleagues noted that two patients with spinal tumours had claudication symptoms, and they had a pre-existing spinal stenosis at a second level[19].

If the lumbar spine is stenotic at two levels, with pressures above venous pressure, the intervening segment of the cauda equina will be congested with venous blood. The extra dural veins will be able to drain into the vertebral venous plexus, but the veins of the cauda equina have no anastomosis, and will become congested.

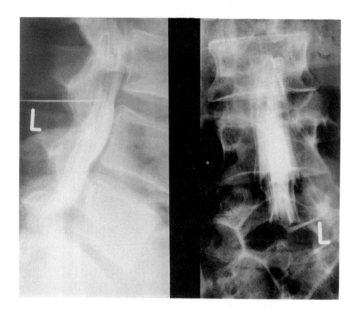

Figure 3. Radiculogram showing a massive disc extrusion occluding the canal. There were no symptoms of claudication.

There is some evidence that the veins of the cauda equina are protected from venous hypertension. There is a physiological valve at the junction where the intradural radicular vein drains centrifugally into the extradural radicular vein. Crock observed that he could not successfully inject contrast against this flow[20], and concluded that there was a physiological valve at this site. Hypertension in the extradural veins is not transmitted to the radicular veins. However in the presence of two levels of central canal stenosis, the radicular veins become engorged.

Experimental studies with a single level compression at 10 mmHg caused little effect in porcine cauda equina, but a two level compression at the same pressure resulted in reduction in axon transport, and nerve conduction[21]. Myeloscopy also shows congested cauda equina in the claudicating patient[22].

Two levels of stenosis in the central canal will congest all the roots of the cauda equina between the compression sites. A single level central stenosis and a more distal root canal stenosis would congest a single root. This might explain the mechanism of unilateral claudication (Figure 6). The symmetrical displacement of a degenerative spondylolisthesis with a second level of central stenosis will cause bilateral claudication. If the degeneration is asymmetrical as in a degenerative scoliosis, unilateral root claudication is more common[10].

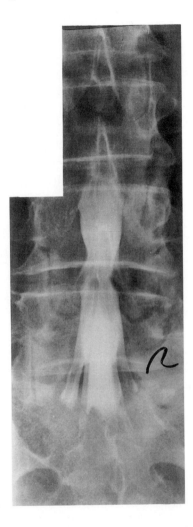

Figure 4. Radiculogram of a patient with unilateral claudication. There is a central canal stenosis at L4/5 and a second level of stenosis from degenerative change affecting the S1 root in the root canal at L5/S1.

10. The dynamics of walking

Claudication is related to the activity of walking. The symptoms do not occur at rest. Thus if venous congestion is important, why do some patients not have rest pain?

We have conducted studies of the porcine cauda equina using the model of Olmarker

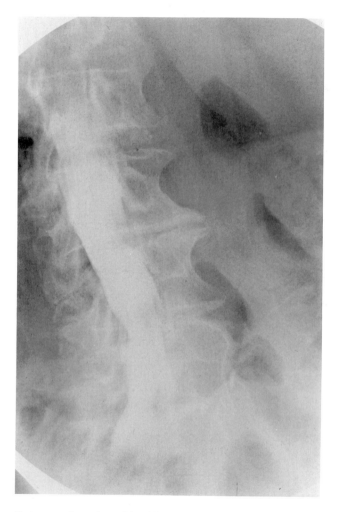

Figure 5. A radiculogram of a patient with unilateral claudication showing gross degenerative lumbar scoliosis, and partial occlusion at L4/5 levels. There was root canal stenosis at L5/S1.

and Rydevik[21], measuring the blood flow with laser doppler (Figure 7). We observed[23] that by stimulating the cauda equina electrically, the blood flow increased rapidly to 300% of the resting level. This was maintained during 30 minutes of stimulation. When applying a low level of compression (10 mmHg) at a single level, there was little change in blood flow. Electrical stimulation of the proximal cauda equina caused a large and

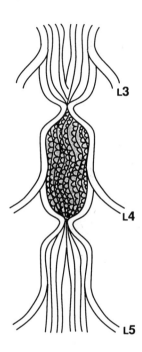 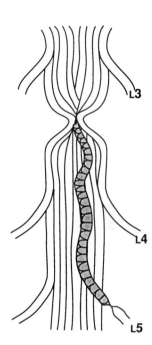

Figure 6. Diagram to show how a double level low pressure central canal stenosis will cause venous congestion of all the roots of the cauda equina between the blocks. The arterioles will supply blood to the roots, but venous pressure will build up to the level of the block pressure. With a single level central stenosis and a more distal root canal stenosis, one root will become congested.claudication.

sustained rise in blood flow. However when applying a double level low pressure compression at 10 mmHg, the flow in the intervening segment fell to 36% of the resting flow. Then when stimulating the cauda equina proximally, there was a sluggish rise in flow to 200% above resting flow, followed in a few minutes by a fall to 40% of the resting flow. The increased flow was therefore not maintained.

If this phenomenon occurs in patients with a double level spinal stenosis, then claudication may be the result of a failure of sustained rise in blood flow when the congested nerve roots are stimulated. We suggest that the increase in flow with electrical stimulation is a result of arterial vasodilatation, and that this usually occurs when walking. There is probably a failure of this arterial vasodilatation in the presence of venous congestion, causing the symptoms of neurogenic claudication. There is a failure of motor activity in the legs.

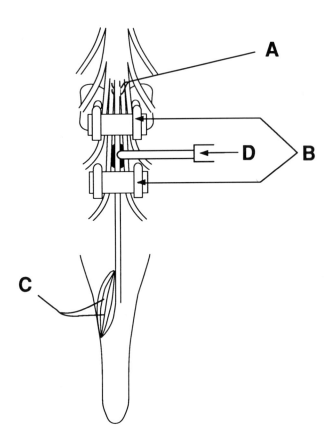

Figure 7. Diagram showing a double level occlusion of the porcine cauda equina at low pressure (2 kPa) (B). The blood flow in the cauda equina was measured by laser doppler (D). Electrical stimulation was applied proximately (A), and tail muscle EMG recording obtained (C).

An arterial component to the pathophysiology of neurogenic claudication would explain the common association between this condition and peripheral vascular disease. It would explain also the observation that neurogenic claudication generally occurs only in the arterio-sclerotic age group. It might explain why some patients respond to calcitonin, which has a powerful arteriolar vasodilation effect.

Furthermore the activity of walking increases the blood flow in the cauda equina which will increase the effective block pressure at the site of the stenosis. Secondly, there will be a rise in the extradural venous pressure, as the extradural veins dilate in response to the exercising lower limbs. Finally the rotatory effect on the spinal segments when walking will reduce the available space in the vertebral canal, particularly in the root canal, where the capsule of the facet joints limit the space for the nerve root complex.

11. Where is the nociceptive source?

Patients have difficulty in describing the symptoms of neurogenic claudication. Some complain of weakness and tiredness, suggesting that there may be a failure of motor activity. Others have pain and cramp similar to the pain of intermittent claudication.

We have postulated that there may be a reflex arc between the proprioceptor in the lower limbs, through the cauda equina to the cord, and then down to L2, to the sympathetic chain and then to the muscle vessels in the lower limb (Figure 8). We suggest that the muscle arterioles which dilate with sympathetic activity, fail to dilate if this reflex arc is blocked. Thus if the cauda equina is congested with venous blood, the reflex arc is interrupted, and the normal vasodilation of the muscle vessels as a result of sympathetic activity fails. The vessels can partially dilate in response to metabolites, but this is incomplete.

We have therefore used Positron Emission Tomography (PET) to measure the blood flow in the muscles of the lower limbs in patients with unilateral neurogenic claudication. We found a mixed response[24]. One patient with spinal stenosis, and normal peripheral vessels had a poor vasodilatation response to exercise in the symptomatic limb. However two other patients with unilateral claudication had similar vascular responses in both limbs, which was not compatible with our hypothesis. It will require a larger study to determine whether a blocked reflex arc is important in some patients with neurogenic claudication. It is probable that we are dealing with a heterogenous problem, with some patients experiencing root pain, others root dysfunction, and others ischaemic muscle pain.

12. Summary

The evidence to date suggests that neurogenic claudication occurs when there is a double level low pressure stenosis. A two level central stenosis tends to be associated with bilateral claudication. A central stenosis and a more distal root canal stenosis is associated with unilateral claudication. There are no symptoms at rest. However during the activity of walking the normal vasodilatory response fails, and with this failure there is impaired nerve conduction, producing the leg symptoms. This is compounded by the activity of walking when the stenosis pressure rises from (a) arterial vasodilatation within the dura, (b) a rise in extradural venous pressure, and (c) the mechanical rotatory effect of walking. Arteriosclerosis probably contributes to the failed arterial response in this syndrome.

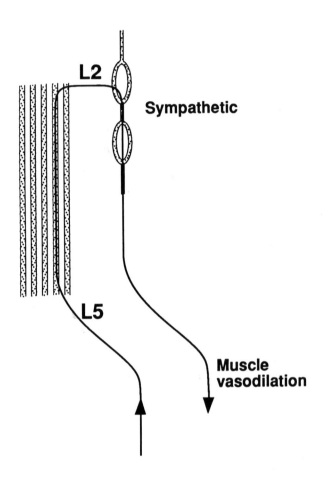

Figure 8. Diagram of a possible reflex arc from the proprioceptor in the lower limb, through the cauda equina and out at L2 to the sympathetic chain, resulting in vasodilatation of the muscle arterioles.

13. References

1.   J. DeJerine, *Press Med.* **19** (1911) 981.
2.   C. Van Gelderen, *Acta Psychatr. Neurol.* **23** (1948) 57-68.
3.   Bermark, 1950. *Acta Med. Scand.* **246** (Suppl) (1950) 30.

4.   H. Verbiest, *J. Bone Joint Surg.* **36-B** (1954) 230.
5.   J.E. Johansson, T.W. Barrington, M. Amelie, *Spine* **7** (1982) 150-158.
6.   G.X. Dong, R.W. Porter, *Spine* **14** (1989) 965-969.
7.   S.D. Boden, D.O. Davis, T.S. Dina, N.J. Patronas, S.W. Wiesel, *J. Bone Joint Surg.* **72-A** (1990) 403-408.
8.   N.R. Schonstron, J.H. Hansson, *Clinical Biomechanics* **6** (1991) 19-24.
9.   A. Kurihara, Y. Tanaka, N. Tsumura, Y. Iwasaki, *Spine* **13** (1988) 1308.
10.   R.W. Porter, D. Ward, *Spine* **17** (1992) 9-15.
11.   K. Olmarker, *Acta Orthop. Scand.* **Supplement 242** (1991) 62.
12.   B.L. Rydevik, R.A. Pedowitz, A.R. Hargens, M.R. Swenson, R.R. Myers, S.R. Garfin, *Spine* **16** (1991) 487-493.
13.   R.B. Delamarter, H.H. Bohlman, L.D. Dodge, C. Biro, *J. Bone Joint Surg.* **72A** (1990) 110-120.
14.   A. Naylor, *J. Bone Joint Surg.* **61-B** (1990) 306-309.
15.   K. Bose, P. Balasybramanian, *Spine* **9** (1984) 16-18.
16.   L. Ciric, A. Michael, M.D. Mikhael, J.A. Tarkington, N.A. Vick, *J. Neuro Surg.* **53** (1980) 433-443.
17.   W.H. Kirkaldy-Willis, T.H. Wedge, K. Yang-Hing, S. Tehnag, V. De Korompay, R. Shennon, *Clin. Orth.* **169** (1982) 171-178.
18.   F. Postacchini, *Lumbar Spine Stenosis* (Springer-Verlag, New York, 1988) p.141.
19.   R.A. McGuire, M.D. Brown, B.A. Green, *Spine* **12** (1987) 1062-1066.
20.   M.V. Crock, M. Yamagaishi, M.C. Crock, *Springer-Verlag*, Vienna (1986)
21.   K. Olmarker, S. Holm, B. Rydevik, *Clin. Orthop.* **279** (1992) 35-39.
22.   Y. Ooi, F. Mita, Y. Satoh, 1990, *Spine* **15** (1990) 544-549.
23.   A.R. Baker, T.A. Collins, R.W. Porter, C. Kidd, *Spine* (1994) (in press).
24.   G.F. Keenan, G.P. Ashcroft, G.H. Roditi, N.T. Evans, R.W. Porter, *Spine* (1994) (in press).

CHAPTER 14

THE ROLE OF VASCULAR DAMAGE IN THE DEVELOPMENT OF NERVE ROOT PROBLEMS

M.I.V. Jayson and A.J. Freemont

1. Introduction

Most back problems are due to mechanical disorders. In many cases it is difficult to identify the specific mechanical problems although in some patients disorders such as herniated intervertebral disc, spondylolisthesis or spinal stenosis may be identified. Commonly however the clinical pattern relates poorly to the objective evidence of mechanical damage. Some patients with advanced degenerative change may be symptom free and others with minimal symptoms experience severe and widespread symptoms. Plain x-rays[1] and MRI scans[2] correlate only poorly with the presence of back symptoms. Resolution of nerve root pain can occur despite persisting nerve root pressure.

Commonly mechanical back symptoms fluctuate. Patients develop acute episodes of pain which then remit. They may remain symptom free or have only minor problems until the next acute episode. However the degenerative change in the spine will be there throughout. It is clear that there are other features which are present and playing a role in causing the presence of symptoms.

In this review we will be describing the roles of vascular damage, fibrosis and chronic inflammation in association with mechanical disorders of the spine and their relevance to back symptoms.

Ankylosing spondylitis is a chronic inflammatory disorder involving the spine. It leads to a characteristic history of pain and stiffness which is aggravated by rest and relieved by exercise. Many patients with mechanical back problems provide a similar history. It is not uncommon to develop a lot of aching and stiffness in bed and stiffness when the patient first wakes up or which develops with prolonged sitting in a chair. Relief is obtained by getting up and doing some exercise. For these patients anti-inflammatory drugs appear particularly effective. The work we have undertaken suggests that venous obstruction and engorgement occur in association with mechanical damage and the static posture is likely to aggravate this. Moving around can improve venous return and reduce venous hypertension. The pattern of symptoms is remarkably similar to that in people with varicose veins. Standing still aggravates the problem and moving around and exercise improves venous drainage and provides relief.

At operation a layer of granulation tissue is often observed around the margin of a prolapse. This is most marked when the disc rupture is complete to the outer border of the annulus fibrosus. Enhanced CT scans or MRI scans may demonstrate this as an enhancing area at the edge of a prolapse[6] and is thought to be due to increased blood volume in this area reflecting increased vascularity. On radiculography in patients with herniated intervertebral discs there may be swelling of the affected nerve root indicating oedema.

Adhesions are commonly found around nerve roots. On histological examination. There is hyperplasia of the perineurium and chronic inflammatory cell infiltration[7].

Similar changes may be found around damaged nerve roots in spinal stenosis[8]. On experimental disc prolapse in animals[9] there is an initial inflammatory reaction with granulation tissue which later becomes more fibrous. These studies suggest that there is commonly a tissue reaction to mechanical damage which in turn may affect the nerve root. The nature of this tissue reaction is subject to much debate.

Although an inflammatory role for herniated nucleus pulposus has been suggested[10] our own observations suggest that in spines in which there has not been any form of previous intervention the pathological changes are vascular damage and fibrosis but without inflammatory cell infiltration. Only when there has been some previous invasive procedure such as previous surgery or oil based myelography can inflammatory cells be found and then the fibrosis may be much more exuberant.

2. Fibrinolytic studies in association with spine problems

Fibrinogen is normally present in the blood. Polymerisation to form a fibrin clot is a normal physiological response to tissue damage. The clot stops blood leaking from damaged blood vessels. In time the fibrinolytic system is activated. This is a complex cascade of reactions in which fibrin is cleaved by plasmin to form fibrin degradation products. Plasmin is formed from plasminogen which has been activated by tissue plasminogen activator. The whole system is inhibited by tissue plasminogen activator inhibitor. Excess of the inhibitor will cause a defect in fibrinolytic activity.

Following trauma there is normally a temporary decrease in fibrinolytic activity which then gradually returns to normal over the succeeding weeks. This means that the clearance of the fibrin clot will only occur relatively slowly giving the tissues a chance of heal. Eventually the clot will clear and blood vessels will return to normal. A prolonged defect in fibrinolytic activity may be associated with a failure to clear fibrin and may interfere with the diffusion of oxygen and nutrients in tissues and be responsible for the development of chronic tissue damage[11].

We have studied the fibrinolytic activity in patients with chronic back pain. We have found that there is a decrease in fibrinolytic activity as compared with control subjects and it is most severe in patients with particularly bad back problems such as arachnoiditis although there were similar trends in other groups of back pain patients[12]. The particular abnormalities found are a significant increase in the euglobulin clot lysis time and a decrease in fibrin plate lysis area. These functional changes appear due to an excess of tissue plasminogen activator inhibitor[13].

This can in part explain why the radiographs correlate poorly with back problems. We have compared patients with similar degrees of degenerative change in the spine in subjects with and without back pain and found that the fibrinolytic defect correlates with the presence of symptoms. We have followed patients presenting with their first episodes of back pain and sciatica and followed them over a period of one year. The changes in fibrinolytic activity correlate with clinical outcome with those patients who failed to resolve having a persistent defect[14]. However these fibrinolytic changes correlate very poorly with individual clinical or imaging features[12].

These findings suggest that changes in fibrinolytic activity can be an objective markers of the severity of the back problem although they are not present in all back pain subjects. We believe they reflect the vascular changes we describe. They could act as a secondary pathogenic mechanism so that failure to clear fibrin can contribute towards the persistence of tissue damage. In this context defective fibrinolytic activity has been identified as an adverse prognostic marker in patients undergoing spine surgery[14]. This is in keeping with the fibrinolytic defect being a marker of the vascular damage and possibly playing a secondary pathogenic role.

These changes may also explain why smoking is a risk factor for spine problems[15-16]. Smoking is associated with a defective fibrinolytic system[17]. This may explain the development of chronic vascular disease and its association with spine disorders.

Studies have been undertaken of fibrinolytic enhancement using Stanozolol which is an anabolic steroid of relatively low virilising potential. In a pilot study[18] we found it was helpful for less severe chronic back problems but we failed to find any benefit in the more severe post-surgical cases[19] despite normalising fibrinolytic activity. We believe the most probable explanation is that in these subjects vascular damage has already taken place so the chances of benefit are likely to be small. When fibrinolytic therapy with tissue plasminogen activator is used for coronary thrombosis it is only effective if administered within a few hours of coronary artery obstruction. Delayed treatment is of no value. Similar mechanisms may well operate in the spine. In these patients the vascular obstruction and ischaemic damage is long standing and not reversible by fibrinolytic enhancement.

3. Experimental studies

An elegant series of studies have been performed in animal models determining how graded compression on nerve roots effects their structure and function. These studies were performed on the pig cauda equina as it resembles the human cauda equina in various respects.

An inflatable balloon was placed across the cauda equina and the effects of varying pressures on the neural and vascular anatomy, nerve root blood flow and nerve conduction were determined[20]. Minor compression of the nerve roots of the order of 5-10 mmHg would induce venous congestion in the intra-neural microcirculation[21]. Greater pressures in the order of 50 mmHg induced oedema formation[22]. This was more marked when pressures were applied rapidly. With pressures of 50-75 mmHg there were changes in both afferent and efferent nerve conduction[23].

The vascular supply to the peripheral nerves differs from that to the nerve roots. In the peripheral nerves there is a much more developed arteriolar and venular network than in the nerve roots. Also in the nerve roots the main vessels are much more superficial and more easily exposed to mechanical deformation with no regional arteriolar blood supply[24]. As a result the nerve roots are at a much greater risk of vascular obstruction due to mechanical compression.

These findings all indicate that nerve root compression even at low pressures can cause vascular obstruction oedema formation and impairment of neurological function. This pathogenic sequence is similar to those found in our own observations in man.

4. Laboratory studies

We have been involved in two major studies investigating the role of vascular changes, inflammation and intra-neural fibrosis and neural atrophy in the pathogenesis of nerve root damage.

4.1. Cadaveric studies

We undertook a study on a series of 125 cadavers. 25 of these were from patients who had long-standing back pain of more than three years. This was documented in their clinical records but in every case had been managed conservatively. 14 had undergone previous myelography. All 25 had died from conditions unrelated to back pain. The other 100 specimens were from a sequential group of patients who came to autopsy following sudden death. Most commonly they had died from myocardial infarction, pulmonary embolism or acute intracranial haemorrhage. Sequential cases were studied in this control group with the proviso that there was no previous history of venous hypertension, endocrine disease, spine instrumentation or documented history of back pain sufficient to have caused them to see their General Practitioner or a Hospital Specialist.

The lumbo-sacral spine was removed and fixed in neutral buffered formalin. It was then cut longitudinally and tissue blocks incorporating the intervertebral root canal and the hemisected spinal canal were taken from alternate sides from L1/2 to L5/S1 (Figure 1). The blocks were classified and serially sectioned. Histological analyses were performed and the area of the intervertebral nerve root canal occupied by the nerve complex and the veins was calculated by histomorphometric analysis (Figure 2). The proportion of the nerve root occupied by fibrous tissue and neural tissue was also determined.

There were little differences between the changes to be seen in the 25 back pain patients or the 100 control specimens. Disc bulging or frank sequestration was found commonly being present in 59 per cent of the back pain group and 41 per cent of the levels in the control group. The protruding disc impinged on vascular structures or fat within the intervertebral root canal and spinal canal (Figures 3 and 4) but only in the most severe sequestrations and usually associated with massive osteophyte formation was nerve root compression observed (Figure 5). Vascular compression in the lower part of the intervertebral root canal was always associated with prominent dilatation of the vessels of the vessels of the venous plexus in the intervertebral root canal and fibrosis within and around the spinal nerve and nerve roots. There was a direct significant statistical relationship between the amount of venous dilatation and the proportion of the nerve root occupied by perineural and intraneural fibrous tissue (Figure 6).

We also found changes in the soft tissues around the nerve root. The fat cells that occupy the majority of the intervertebral root canal show the changes associated with early fat necrosis. The microvessels around the nerve root have extensive thickening of their basement membranes (Figure 7). Where the meninges cover the nerve roots there is proliferation of the arachnoid cells and formation of psammoma bodies[25]. These three changes are characteristic of ischaemic damage.

Disc bulging and sequestration were always associated with degenerative change in the disc. Typically they included chondrocyte proliferation and myxoid change in the

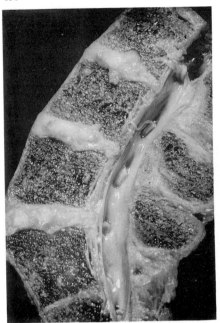

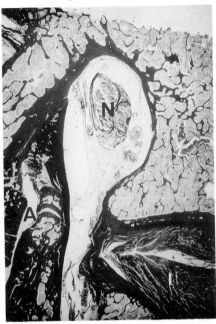

Figure 1. Macroscopic view of normal disc

Figure 2. Histological section of a normal intervertebral root canal showing the relationship between the intervertebral disc (I), apophyseal joint (A) and the nerve root (N).

matrix. The disc frequently contained propagated intra-discal fissures which were cracks and splits running through the disc and usually entering into and through the posterior annulus where they turned caudally to end at the vertebral end plate adjacent to the vertebral rim. In these cases commonly there was damage to the vertebral end plate which could be seen as defects in the cartilage and bone (Figure 8). Through these defects there were new vascular channels accompanied by neural ingrowth extending into the disc and propagating along the edges of the fissures (Figure 9). Elsewhere within the biopsies high densities of nerves were found in the longitudinal and intraspinous ligaments, the periosteum on the vertebrae and the walls of the epidural and peridural veins.

It was common to find fibrin deposition within the dilated vascular channels in the intervertebral root canals (Figure 10). In places there was occlusive thrombus formation showing organisation which is absolute evidence that the thrombus had formed prior to death[26] (Figure 11).

There were no obvious differences between the type or extent of pathological changes at any one level between the symptomatic and asymptomatic individuals. However when the changes described were analysed over all five levels from each spine important differences emerged.

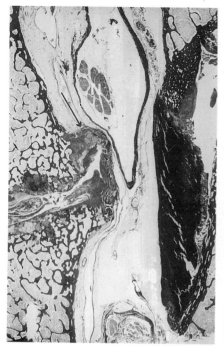

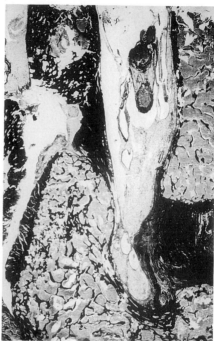

Figure 3. An osteophyte associated with discal extrusion. The neural element (N) is not impinged upon but the local venous channels are completely compressed by the extruded tissue and osteophytic bone (arrowed).

Figure 4. This discal protrusion is associated with venous compression, perineural fibrosis and changes in the fat within the IVRC seen elsewhere in sites of poor tissue oxygenation.

Discal pathology (distal protrusion or sequestration) was found in 96 per cent of symptomatic cases compared with 23 per cent of asymptomatic cases; venous dilatation in 96 per cent compared with 47 per cent; multiple venous dilatation in 48 per cent compared to 6 per cent; peri-radicular fibrosis in 100 per cent compared with 32 per cent; intra-radicular fibrosis in 84 per cent compared with 12 per cent; organising thrombus in 16 per cent compared with 5 per cent.

Overall the proportion of the area of the intervertebral canal occupied by dilated veins was 28.8 ± 5.9 per cent in symptomatic patients and 10.6 ± 3.8 per cent in asymptomatic patients ($P < 0.001$). The proportion of the nerve root occupied by fibrous tissue was 35.1 ± 7.2 per cent in symptomatic patients and 14.8 ± 6.6 per cent in asymptomatic patients ($P < 0.005$).

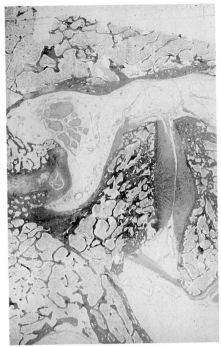

Figure 5. An example of a large discal protrusion and associated osteophyte formation in which there is impingement upon the neural complex.

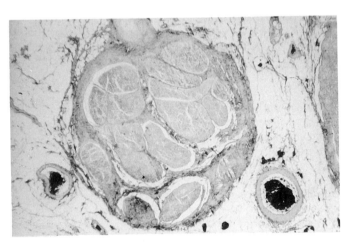

Figure 6. Peri- and intra-neural fibrosis extends beyond the intradural nerve roots.

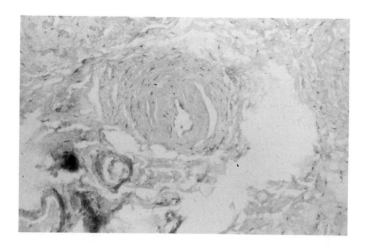

Figure 7. Within the nerve there is extensive thickening of the basement membrane of the microvasculature. This may contribute to the tissue ischaemia.

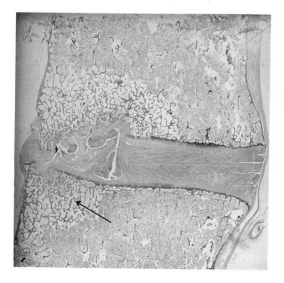

Figure 8. Discal injury leads to profound changes in the cartilaginous endplate and adjacent marrow. In this figure the bony endplate is also disrupted and there has been local loss of haemopoietic marrow (arrowed).

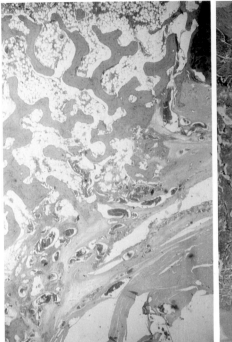 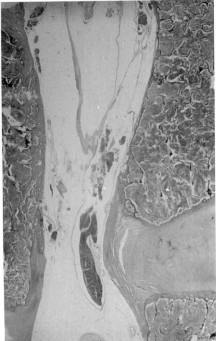

Figure 9. Relatively minor injury to the endplate results in the ingrowth into the disc of blood vessels and nerves arising from the medullary cavity of the bone.

Figure 10. This vessel adjacent to a small extrusion contains thrombus.

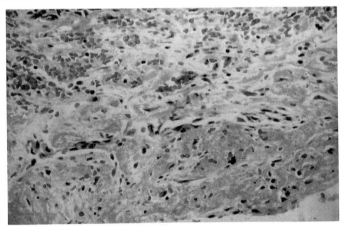

Figure 11. The thrombus is undergoing organisation indicating that the thrombotic events occurred prior to death.

We conclude from these observations:-

1.   Disc and associated pathologies are not necessarily associated with significant back pain.
2.   The greater the numbers of spinal levels affected the greater the probability of back pain.
3.   Extensive vascular changes accompany this pathology. These include venous dilatation and thromboses; extensive ingrowth of vessels; thickening of the basement membranes of the capillaries and venules.
4.   Morphological changes indicative of tissue ischaemia accompany the discal and vascular changes.
5.   Venous dilatation in the intervertebral root canal is linked with peri-radicular and inter-radicular fibrosis.

4.2. Biopsy studies

In order to relate the cadaveric observations to studies in life we undertook histological and *in-situ* cell and molecular biology observations on biopsies taken from peri-radicular structures at the time of primary spinal surgery for mechanical spinal disease. These biopsies included vascular, fibrous and adipose tissue. In order to obtain control material we examined peri-radicular tissue excised from 'fresh' cadavers obtained within 4 hours of death and also similar specimens excised from organ donors at the time of organ donation[27].

At the morphological level the surgical specimens obtained from the back subjects showed tissue fibrosis, fibrin deposition, endothelial vasculation and neovascularisation which was not found in the control material.

The two tissue probing techniques of immunohistochemistry and in situ hybridisation were used to explore the cell and molecular biology of the vessels and connective tissues within the intervertebral root canal. Studies of von Willebrand Factor (vWF) which is a product of endothelial cells and whose release is associated with platelet aggregation and thrombus formation showed loss of vWF but increase in mRNA in the endothelial cells of the operated group. vWF is normally stored in the endothelial cell cytoplasm within organelles called Wiebel-Palade bodies. When the endothelial cell is stimulated the vWF is discharged and no longer immunodetectable. If stimulation continues vWF mRNA is unregulated increasing the detectable in situ hybridisation signal but because the gene product is continuously secreted insufficient is available to be detected immunohistochemically within the cell. It therefore appears that in the symptomatic patient with mechanical spine disease the venous channels around the nerve root are subject to endothelial cell stimulation leading to release of vWF which in turn causes platelet aggregation and thrombosis. Up-regulation of vWF mRNA was associated with intravascular accumulation of platelets which we could demonstrate by the presence of platelet glycoprotein IIa. There were other changes in endothelial function in the operated group of patients. These include endothelial cell expression of the fibrogenic cytokines IL-1 and TGF-β. Fibroblasts within the fibrous tissue surrounding these vessels showed a marked increase in mRNA for Type I collagen. Although we could not quantify the absolute amount of protein or mRNA the relative staining of densities suggested that the increase in Type I collagen mRNA was directly proportional to the level of cytokine expression.

Both morphological studies and histochemical probing of the tissue with antibodies directed towards the cell surface antigens expressed on B lymphocytes, T lymphocyte subsets, macrophages and mast cells failed to reveal an inflammatory cell infiltrate in any specimen.

5. A unifying hypothesis to explain these findings

The principal conclusion of our studies relates to vascular changes with peri-radicular fibrosis. The data indicate that degenerative change in the spine with disc disease leads to venous compression in the lower part of the intervertebral root canal and disturbed blood flow. Particularly in multi-level disease significant impairment of venous blood flow from occurs leading to venous hypertension manifest as venous dilatation. The poor blood flow causes tissue ischaemia, endothelial dysfunction and thrombus formation in the vessels of the intervertebral root canal. Simultaneously changes in endothelial function lead to the synthesis of fibrinogenic cytokines. The contribution of new cytokine synthesis and tissue ischaemia results in increased collagen synthesis by local fibroblasts.

At the same time the trauma that causes disc disease results in morphological evidence of discal and para-discal tissue disruption. This leads to an attempted repair process in which new blood vessels grow into the disc. These vessels secrete matrix degrading enzymes which further weaken the discal connective tissues and are also accompanied by nerves. There is a potential cycle of persistent or increasing tissue damage and potential pain induction.

6. Possible association between clinical observations, pathological appearances and back pain

It is commonly proposed that direct nerve root compression causes pain. In acute disc prolapse this is clearly the case but we have been unable to find any significant association between chronic pain and direct nerve root compression.

Inflammation has also been implicated in the genesis of pain. Again there may be evidence of this in acute disc herniation in which herniated nuclear material can be inflammogenic but in neither cadaveric nor biopsy studies were we able to identify any conventional inflammatory cell infiltrate on morphological or immunohistochemical analysis of the soft tissues within the spine and nerve root canal. Our observations suggest that the redness in the peridural tissues and annulus often noticed at surgery for chronic disc herniation and reported as inflammation is not inflammation as such but rather due to the appearances of vascular dilatation.

In addition to nerves penetrating the disc which would be prone to physical stimulation our investigations suggest another potential mechanism by which nerves could be stimulated in spinal disease. Dense aggregates of nerves are distributed around the peri-radicular veins and associated with vessels associated with the traumatised and degenerative discs. They show evidence of platelet aggregation and thrombus formation and the surrounding tissues demonstrate features associated with ischaemia. The nociceptive nerve endings could be stimulated by a variety of chemical mediators including kinins, 5-hydroxytryptamine, prostanoids, lactic acid and potassium ions. In the context of our observations of blood vessels and the distribution of nerve endings it is interesting to note that kinins are formed during coagulation, 5-hydroxytryptamine is released from activated aggregated platelets and prostanoids and lactic acid and potassium ions are released from ischaemic cells.

7. Future work

Clearly there is a number of different mechanisms of back pain. Our studies highlight how modern investigation techniques can be employed to provide a better understanding of the tissue changes that develop. In particular they indicate the importance of disturbed vascular physiology which can lead to secondary ischaemia and fibrosis and also play a potential role in the cycle leading to further disc degeneration. Treatment aimed at normalising endothelial function and maintaining intravascular flow may well prevent the development of these chronic problems although it is clear that this strategy would have to be started early in the course of the disease.

8. References

1. J.S. Lawrence, in *Rheumatism in Population*, (Heinemann, 1977) 68.
2. G. Buirski, M. Silbertstein, *Spine* **18** (1993) 1808.
3. S.R. Garfin, B.L. Rydevik and R.A. Brown, *Spine* **16** (1991) 162.
4. I. Goldie, *Acta Pathologica Scandinavica* **42** (1958) 302.
5. C. Hirsch, *J. Bone Joint Surg.* **41-B** (1959) 237.
6. H. Firooznia, I.I. Kricheff, M. Rafii and C. Golimbu, *Neurophysiology* (1963) 221.
7. O. Lindhal and B. Rexed, *Acta Orthop. Scand.* **20** (1951) 215.
8. A. Watanabe and W.W. Parke, *J. Neurosurg.* **64** (1986) 64.
9. H-J. Hansen, *Acta Orthop. Scand.* **Suppl 11** (1952) 1.
10. D. Innes and S. Sevitt, *J. Clin. Path.* **17** (1964) 1.
11. G.D. Pountain, A.L. Keegan and M.I.V. Jayson, *Spine* **12** (1987) 83.
12. R.G. Cooper, W.S. Mitchell, K.J. Illingworth, W. St. Clair Forbes, J.E. Gillespie and M.I.V. Jayson, *Spine* **16** (1991) 1044.
13. P.S. Klimiuk, D.G. Pountain, A.L. Keegan and M.I.V. Jayson, *Spine* **12** (1987) 925.
14. A.K. Haaland, V. Graver, A.E. Ljunggren, M. Loeb, H. Lie, B. Magnaes and H.C. Godal, *Spine* **17** (1992) 1022.
15. M.C. Battié, S.J. Bigos, L.D. Fisher, T.H. Hansson, A.L. Nachemson, D.M. Spengler, M.D. Wortley and J.A. Zeh, *Spine* **14** (1989) 141.

16.   J.W. Frymoyer, M.H. Pope, J.H. Clements, D.G. Wilder, B. MacPherson and T. Ashikaga, *J. Bone Joint Surg.* **65-A** (1983) 213.

17.   T.W. Meade, R. Chakrabarti, A.P. Haines, W.R.S. North and Y. Sterling, *Br. Med. J.* **1** (1979) 153.

18.   W.S. Mitchell, K.J. Illingworth and M.I.V. Jayson, *Br. J. Rheumatol.* **A2** (1988) 12.

19.   R.G. Cooper, M.S. Mitchell, K.J. Illingworth and M.I.V. Jayson, *Scand. J. Rheumatol.* **20** (1991) 414.

20.   K. Olmarker, S. Holm, A-L. Rosenqvist and B. Rydevik, *Spine* **16** (1991) 61.

21.   K. Olmarker, B. Rydevik and S. Holm, *Spine* **14** (1989) 569.

22.   R.A. Pedowitz, S.R. Garfin, J.B. Massie, A.R. Hargens, M.R. Swenson, R.R. Myers and B.L. Rydevik, *Spine* **17** (1992) 194.

23.   B.L. Rydevik, R.A. Pedowitz, A.R. Hargens, M.R. Swenson, R. Myers and S.R. Garfin, *Spine* **16** (1991) 487.

24.   B.L. Rydevik, Etiology of Sciatica in the lumbar spine. Edt. J.N. Weinstein and S.W. Wiesel, (Saunders, 1990) pp.132-145.

25.   J.A. Hoyland and A.J.H. Freemont, *Neuro-orthopaedics* **11** (1991) 83.

26.   J.A. Hoyland, A.J. Freemont and M.I.V. Jayson, *Spine* **14** (1989) 558.

27.   R.G. Cooper, A.J. Freemont, J.A. Hoyland, J.P.R. Jenkins, C.G.H. West, K.J. Illingworth and M.I.V. Jayson, *Spine* In Press.

CHAPTER 15

THE ASSESSMENT OF THE PATIENT WITH LOW BACK PAIN

C.D. Greenough

1. Introduction

Chronic low back pain is now the largest single cause of disability in Western Society. In the United Kingdom (UK) 46% of a randomised sample of the entire population had at one time or another suffered from back pain, and 18% of those reporting pain had had time off work in the preceding year[8]. The cost to the UK National Health Service for treatment of low back pain has been estimated as 1.15 % of the total budget[53]. In 1987 in the United States of America 5.3 million people were disabled due to low back pain and a further 11.7 million had impairment. Compensation and medical costs due to back pain in 1984 were $7.2 billion[13]. This large burden of suffering and its associated high costs have lead to the development of many modalities of treatment within the medical model of health care and in the professions allied to medicine and in a plethora of commercially promoted products. Unfortunately, it remains the case that despite so much available treatment, chronic back pain is an unsolved problem.

The basic unit of the lumbar spine is the motion segment which comprises two adjacent vertebrae together with their intervertebral disc, facet joints, ligaments and muscles. It is in this unit that the source of the pain must lie and it is to this unit that almost all of the current research has been devoted. Unfortunately ever increasing knowledge of the biochemistry and biomechanics of the intervertebral disc and of the anatomy, physiology, biomechanics and pathology of the motion segment together with investigative techniques of ever increasing sophistication have failed to produce significant clinical improvements. When we are dealing with patients with low back pain we must remember that it is not the motion segment which requires treatment but a patient who wants treatment for back pain and its resultant disability.

2. Clinical syndromes

A number of clinical syndromes can be recognised in patients who present with low back pain. Neurogenic claudication, inflammatory diseases and the constellation of symptoms and signs which occur with prolapse of the intervertebral disc are well known. These conditions have specific therapies and are dealt with elsewhere in this volume. The majority of patients, however, present with what is termed 'mechanical low back pain', without neurological involvement. In this regard it is important to remember that referred pain may radiate to the leg and foot[23] so that all pain below the knee is NOT root pain.

Within the broad classification of mechanical low back pain three syndromes may be distinguished. Any combination of these three syndromes may be present in varying degrees in any one individual.

2.1. Discogenic pain

The back 'goes', presenting with episodic acute attacks of low back pain, often with considerable spasm and rigidity of the lumbar spine. It is often triggered off by unguarded movements, particularly in rotation or by minor trauma. The duration of each attack is normally short, of a few days only. Patients often report difficulty with activities requiring rotational movements, such as ironing, hoovering and manoeuvring supermarket trolleys. Examination of these patients in between attacks reveals good or normal spinal movement although there may be an 'extension catch' - an interruption of the normal flow of movement on rising from the flexed position. There is no neurological deficit and tension signs are absent. Radiological examination of these patients is unremarkable with well preserved disc spaces and age related changes only.

2.2. Facet joint pain

These patients present with chronic aching pain, often with radiation into the buttocks and the posterior aspect of the thighs. This pain is made worse after exercise and is associated with stiffness of the spine both in the morning on rising from bed and after prolonged sitting. Stiffness will commonly pass off after half an hour or so. Patients are restless on sitting still. On examination the patient may display limitation of lumbar extension by pain or pain on rising from the flexed position. No hard neurological deficits are found but sometimes motor point tenderness exists. On radiological examination disc spaces may be reduced and posterior element of sclerosis may be observed. Axial examination such as CT scanning demonstrate degenerative change in the facet joint.

2.3. Nerve root irritation

Patients present with non-specific leg pains both during and after activity but this never amounts to neurogenic claudication. They also present vague sensory disturbances and sensation of pins and needles particularly related to activity. Dysaesthetic pain at night may be a feature with burning type of pain on retiring to bed. On examination these patients do not present any definite neurological deficit and spinal movements are normally good. Mild tension signs may be present.

These syndromes are based on medical models of low back pain used in my own practice. Other overlapping syndromes are described in the literature[9] and other practitioners such as osteopaths and chiropractors have their own philosophies of classification. However, the usefulness of a classification rests largely on its ability to predict prognosis and identify the most suitable treatment for a particular case. This has been studied for a similar medical model.

3. A study of low back pain following injury

Greenough[16] in a carefully controlled retrospective study defined a group of 300 patients complaining of low back pain following injury. 150 patients were claiming compensation for their injury and 150 were not. These patients were all treated conservatively and at follow up 274 (91%) patients were reviewed at a median follow up of 50 months (range 13 - 300) for the compensation patients and 52 months (range 9 - 332) for the non compensation patients. The diagnosis (Table 1) was made by a single orthopaedic specialist who treated only spinal conditions and was confirmed by radiological investigations where appropriate.

Table 1. Diagnosis by compensation group

Diagnosis	Comp.	Non comp.	All patients
Disc prolapse	17	28	42 (15%)
Discogenic pain	71	58	129 (45%)
Spondylolisthesis	9	10	19 (7%)
Facet arthropathy	17	26	43 (15%)
Soft tissue strain	21	11	32 (10%)
Other	10	12	22 (8%)

An injury severity score was allocated to each patient. At presentation two psychometric instruments were administered to each patient; the Pain Drawing[39] and the inappropriate signs of Waddell[52]. These were scored according to published criteria and if either of the scores was positive then the patient was defined as disturbed. Social group was allocated from the Ann Daniel Scale[5].

At review each patient completed the Low-Back Outcome Score[18]. Multiple regression analysis was performed using the Outcome Score as the dependent variable with sixteen independent variables. The total variance explained (r^2) was 48.3%. The variables examined and their significance appear in Tables 2 and 3.

Table 2. Factors with a significant influence on outcome

Compensation claim	$P < 0.0001$
Psychological disturbance	$P < 0.002$
Time off work	$P < 0.02$
Age at injury	$P < 0.005$
Sex	$P < 0.02$
Social group	$P < 0.01$
Twisting or jerking injury	$P < 0.05$

Table 3. Factors with no significant influence on outcome

Diagnosis
Severity of injury
Length of follow up
Neurological deficit
Migrant status
Smoking
Interval between injury and initial consultation
Timing of first therapy
Marital status

The two variables of compensation and psychological disturbance at presentation between them accounted for 35 % of the variance, or more than half of the explained variance. It is of interest that the severity of the injury and neurological deficit had no prognostic significance.

Despite the diagnosis being made by a single, experienced practitioner using consistent criteria the diagnostic classification employed could not be shown to be of any prognostic significance. This implies that specific therapies directed to these specific diagnoses are unlikely to prove effective and in fact the results of therapy in this study group have been investigated[19]. A number of therapies including educational classes, exercises, facet injections and epidurals were used and only educational classes could be shown to have a significant effect and then only in a small subset of patients. Interestingly, whereas non compensation patients improved following facet injection compensation patients became worse!

Thus in this carefully constructed population patient related factors outside the control of the treating practitioner had far more influence on the outcome than diagnosis or treatment. This is in accordance with the findings of other workers.

Compensation was first associated with disability when Rigler coined the term 'compensation neurosis' in 1879[36] and a number of studies have suggested that compensation does retard and impair recovery from injury[6,43,50]. Sander and Meyers[43] reported the results of railroad workers, 35 of whom sustained their injury at work, and 30 while off duty. There was no difference in the average age of the two groups (38.4 years and 39.1 years respectively), nor in the injury severity and the length of time off work was not significantly related to the worker's gender. Those injured on duty, however, were off work for a mean of 14.9 months whereas those injured off duty were off work for an average of 3.6 months only. In line with the results of facet joint injections compensation has also been shown elsewhere to influences the results of treatment programmes[25]. These authors studied the response to a rehabilitation programme of 272 compensation claimants and 237 non compensation patients. They found 88.5% of the non compensation group were rated as improved compared with 55.8% of the compensation group. Compensation patients also had significantly more treatments than non compensation patients.

In Greenough's study[16] settlement of the claim was associated with a small increase in the Outcome score in the men, but there was no change in reported pain and no improvement in employment status or psychological disturbance. Similar findings have been reported by several other workers[29,48,49] in contrast to the older work by Miller[31,32] who had claimed that legal claimants lost their psychological symptoms and returned to work shortly after settlement. Further, Greenough demonstrated that following settlement the patients seeking treatment were more likely to have psychological disturbance than those not seeking treatment. As the response to therapy in compensation patients depends in part on the extent of psychological disturbance[7], this has important implications if operation is contemplated. In addition compensation has been found to reduce the response of psychological disturbance itself to treatment[50].

Psychological disturbance has been noted in many patients following back injuries[6,30,51] and has been shown to reduce the response of patients with low back pain to conservative therapy[1], chemonucleolysis[55] and surgery[37]. A relationship between psychological disturbance and litigation has been proposed, although the incidence varies with the framework of the observer[31,32,36,40].

Greenough found twisting, slipping and jerking injuries produced more disability than other injuries, a finding in agreement with other studies[24,26,28,33]. These differences, however, were not observed in the non compensation patients. This suggests that it may not be the mechanism of the injury but some other factor which was associated with the reduction in the outcome score. Slipping and jerking accidents, for example slipping on an oil spillage on the floor, may be more demonstrably the fault of a third party.

Social group has been previously observed to exert an influence on recovery and migrant status has been shown not to affect outcome after controlling for social group[21].

The lack of prognostic significance of an initial neurological deficit (defined in Greenough's study as the loss of a reflex or the weakness of a specific muscle group) agrees with the findings of Currey *et al.*[4]. If such 'hard' examination findings are not of prognostic value then it may be unwise to rely on less definite signs such as flexion, which is known to be influenced by psychological disturbance[38].

Educational classes appeared to be of value, a finding also noted by Berquist-Ullman and Larsson[2] and Sikorski[44]. More specific treatments could not be shown to be effective which is perhaps un-surprising in view of the lack of influence of diagnosis.

Similar findings have been observed in fusion surgery for low back pain. Greenough *et al.* have reported the results of one hundred and fifty one consecutive patients undergoing anterior interbody lumbar spinal fusion for intractable back pain[20]. There were seventy seven men (median age 40 (17 - 57)) and seventy four women (median age 42 (20 - 62)). Sixty four men and forty two women were claiming compensation for a back injury or for occupational back pain. The indications for surgery were discogenic or mechanical back pain in 95 patients, failed previous surgery in 34 patients, motion segment instability in 4 patients and spondylolysis or spondylolisthesis in 14 patients. The distribution of indications was the same between the compensation patients and the non compensation patients. Using the pain drawing[39] and the inappropriate signs of Waddell[52], of the 119 patients with measurable drawings 51 (43 %) were disturbed at presentation.

4. Outcome of treatment

Fusion was performed at a single level in 87 patients, at two levels in 63 patients and at three levels in one patient. The operation was performed through a retroperitoneal approach[11] according to the technique of Crock[3].
Review was undertaken at a minimum two years follow up with a median follow up of 39 (24 - 82) months for the men and 40 (24 - 75) months for the women. 136 patients (90.1 %) were reviewed. The patient completed a satisfaction rating on a four point scale. Disability was assessed using the Low-back Outcome Score[18].
A solid bony fusion was obtained in 76 % of patients. The method of outcome assessment profoundly affected the results; whereas 68 % of patients rated themselves as significantly improved by the procedure (Table 4) only 40 % achieved a good or excellent result on the more objective Low Back Outcome Score (Table 5). Pre-operatively 115 patients were unemployed, whereas at final review 58 were unemployed.

Table 4. Subjective opinions at review

	Compensation Number (%)	Non Compensation Number (%)	All Patients Number (%)
Almost complete relief	15 (18%)	15 (38%)	30 (24%)
Good deal of relief	38 (45%)	16 (41%)	54 (44%)
Only a little relief	23 (27%)	4 (10%)	27 (22%)
No relief or worse	9 (10%)	4 (10%)	13 (10%)

P < 0.05 (Chi-Square)

Table 5. Low back Outcome scores at review

		Compensation Number (%)	Non Compensation Number (%)	All Patients Number (%)
Excellent	(65-75)	8 (10%)	13 (43%)	21 (17%)
Good	(50-64)	19 (22%)	10 (25%)	29 (23%)
Fair	(30-49)	34 (40%)	10 (25%)	44 (35%)
Poor	(0-29)	24 (28%)	7 (17%)	31 (25%)

P < 0.01 (Chi-Square)

Those patients with radiological fusion were not improved compared with those with a pseudarthrosis (Table 6).

Table 6. Effect on Low-back Outcome Score, Patient Satisfaction Rating and reported pain at review of radiological fusion. Median (range, n)

	Fused	Not Fused	P value
Outcome	46 (1-75, 52)	43 (19-75, 15)	ns
Satisfaction	2 (0-3, 53)	2 (0-3, 16)	ns
Pain	4 (0-10, 56)	5 (1-8, 16)	ns

Compensation status and psychological disturbance at presentation were significant prognostic factors (Table 7).

Table 7. Effect on Low-back Outcome Score, Patient Satisfaction Rating and reported pain at review pain of compensation status and pre-operative psychological disturbance. Median (range, n)

	Compensation	Non Compensation	P value
Outcome	42 (1-75, 85)	55 (14-75, 40)	< 0.01
Satisfaction	2 (0-3, 85)	2 (0-3, 39)	< 0.05
Pain	5 (0-10, 89)	3 (0-8, 42)	< 0.05
	Disturbed pre-op	Not disturbed	P value
Outcome	352 (1-75, 46)	47 (14-75, 64)	< 0.05
Satisfaction	2 (0-3, 49)	2 (0-3, 60)	n.s.
Pain	5 (0-10, 50)	4 (0-10, 64)	n.s.

Greenough *et al.*'s finding that radiological fusion is not associated with the outcome in anterior fusion is in agreement with Freebody *et al.*[12] and Flynn and Hoque[10].

Sacks[42] had noted a very powerful association of poor results with the presence of a compensation claim. Stauffer and Coventry[46] reported poor overall results in 83 patients using an objective scoring method with only 32% good results. They also noted a strong association between compensation and poor results; in addition they found an association between pre-operative psychological disturbance and poor results.

Thus the results of a surgical procedure undertaken for low back pain confirm that the prognosis is again heavily influenced by compensation status and to a lesser extent by pre-operative psychological disturbance.

The clinical assessment of the results of spinal surgery is complicated by the large number assessment measures used. Comparison of fourteen different outcome measures in a group of over two hundred patients following lumbar intervertebral disc excision revealed that the proportion of 'successes' was significantly influenced by the outcome measure used, ranging from 97% to 60%[22]. Subjective measures, for example the patients opinion of the operation, gave a higher proportion of 'successful' results when compared to objective measures such as return to original employment. It is also important to recognise that the technical outcome - "has the surgeon achieved what he set out to achieve?" does not necessarily correlate with the clinical result - "Has the patient benefited from the procedure?".

5. Conclusions

In summary initial disability, compensation, psychological distress, socio-economic factors and the assessment technique all have a major role in determining the 'results' of a treatment[15]. Indeed, these factors appear to explain more of the variance of the outcome than the condition or treatment itself. Thus when a practitioner is considering the suitability of a patient for treatment, it is essential that these factors are evaluated. The issue of compensation must be specially explored, a recognised disability score should be completed and patients should complete an appropriate psychometric evaluation.

Greenough & Fraser[17] have presented a review of a number of the psychometric instruments in low back pain. In their study combination techniques were most reliable in identifying psychological distress and a combination of the Modified Somatic Perception Questionnaire[27] and the Zung depression scale[56] was found to be most discriminating.

Our ability to treat low back pain has also been hampered by both the lack of an investigation which will allow the distinction of patients with low back pain from age and sex matched controls and also the lack of an objective outcome measure which does not rely on self report scores or testing over which the patient has some voluntary control. Plain x-rays and flexion and extension views have demonstrated equal numbers of abnormalities in patients with chronic low back pain and in normal age and sex matched volunteers[14,45,47]. Studies of CT scanning have reported similar findings[54]. With the advent of MRI scanning this new technology initially appeared to offer a means of distinguishing patients with low back pain but recently it has become clear that the incidence of abnormalities such as dark discs on MRI is not significantly different between patients and normals.

Recently attention has been draw to a relatively neglected area of the lumbar spine, namely the lumbar musculature. De Luca and associates using an EMG technique were able to show differences in spectral values between groups of rowers with and without back pain[41]. Oliver and Greenough, using a different analysis technique, have been able to demonstrate that EMG analysis of back muscles is reliable from day to day[35]. They were subsequently able to demonstrate that their technique, based on spectral mapping, was able to discriminate patients with low back pain from normal age and sex matched volunteers with a specificity and sensitivity of approximately 80 percent[34]. This technique was relatively load independent and thus was independent of patients voluntary control. Their results fell onto a continuous spectrum with highly trained athletes at one end and chronically disabled low back pain patients at the other. Further work is continuing with long term follow-up studies of volunteers of patients to assess the correlation between changes in clinical conditions and changes in the EMG pattern. If such correlations do exist then this technique may represent a method of objective assessment of patients with low back pain and of monitoring results of treatment.

At the present time the study of the EMG of the spinal muscles is the only technique that has been able to demonstrate measurable differences between back pain patients and normal volunteers and thus at least holds out some hope of future progress in this difficult area.

6. References

1. R.K. Beals and N.W. Hickman, *J. Bone Joint Surg.* **54-A** (1972) 1593.
2. M. Bergquist-Ullman and U. Larsson, *Acta. Orthop. Scand.* **Supp. 170** (1977) 1.
3. H.V. Crock, *Clin. Orthop.* **166** (1982) 157.
4. H.L.F. Currey, R.M. Greenwood, G.G. Lloyd and R.S. Murray, *Rheumatol. Rehabil.* **18** (1979) 94.
5. A. Daniel, *Power, Prvilege and Prestige* (Longman Cheshire, Melbourne 1983) 197.
6. R.H. Dworkin, D.S. Handin, D.M. Richlin, L. Brand and C. Vannucci, *Pain* **23** (1985) 49.
7. R.B. Dzioba and N.C. Doxey, *Spine* **9** (1984) 614.
8. J.C.T. Fairbank, In *Back Pain. Methods For Clinical Investigation and Assessment.* Ed. D.W.L. Hukins and R.C. Mulholland (Manchester University Press, 1986) 1.
9. J.C.T. Fairbank and H. Hall, In *The Lumbar Spine* Ed. Weinstein and Wiesel. (WB Saunders, Philadelphia 1990) 88.
10. J.C. Flynn and M.A. Hoque, *J. Bone Joint Surg.* **61-A** (1979) 1143.
11. R.D. Fraser, *J. Bone Joint Surg.* **64-B** (1982) 44.
12. D. Freebody, R. Bendall and R.D. Taylor, *J. Bone Joint Surg.* **53-B** (1971) 617.
13. J.W. Frymoyer and W. Cats-Baril, *Clin. Orthop.* **221** (1987) 89.
14. T.M. Fullenlove and A.J. Williams, *Radiology* **68** (1957) 572.
15. C.G. Greenough, *Act. Orthop. Scand.* **64 (Supp 251)** (1993) 126.
16. C.G. Greenough, *Act. Orthop. Scand.* **64 Supp. 254** (1993) 1.
17. C.G. Greenough and R.D. Fraser, *Spine* **16** (1991) 1068.
18. C.G. Greenough and R.D. Fraser, *Spine* **17** (1992) 36.
19. C.G. Greenough and R.D. Fraser, *Eur. Spine J.* **3** (1994) 22.
20. C.G. Greenough, L.J. Taylor and R.D. Fraser, *Eur. Spine J.* **3** (1994) 225.

21.   D. Hewson, J. Halcrow and C.S. Brown, *Med. J. Austral.* **147** (1987) 280.
22.   J. Howe and J.W. Frymoyer, Spine **10** (1985) 804.
23.   J.H. Kellgren, *Clin. Sci. Mol. Med.* **4** (1939) 35.
24.   J.L. Kelsey, P.B. Githens, A.A. White III, T.R. Holford, S.D. Walter, T. O'Connor, A.M. Ostfeld, U. Weil, W.O. Southwick and J.A. Calogero, *J. Orthop. Res.* **2** (1984) 61.
25.   E.M. Krusen and D.E. Ford, *J. Amer. Med. Ass.* **166** (1958) 1128.
26.   A. Magora, Scand. *J. Rehab. Med.* **5** (1973) 186.
27.   C.J. Main, *J. Psychosom. Res.* **27** (1983) 503.
28.   D.P. Manning and H.S. Shannon, *Spine* **6** (1981) 70.
29.   G. Mendelson, *Med. J. Austral.* **2** (1982) 132.
30.   G. Mendelson, *Pain* **20** (1984) 169.
31.   H. Miller, *Br. Med. J.* (1961) 919.
32.   H. Miller, *Br. Med. J.* (1961) 992.
33.   M. Molumphy, B. Unger, G.M. Jensen and R.B. Lopopolo, *Physical Therapy* **65** (1985) 482.
34.   C.W. Oliver and C.G. Greenough, *J. Bone Joint Surg.* **76-B Supp I** (1994) 44.
35.   C.W. Oliver, R.A. Royal and C.G. Greenough, *J. Bone Joint Surg.* **75-B Supp III** (1993) 246.
36.   N. Parker, *Med. J. Austral.* **2** (1977) 318.
37.   H.C. Pheasant, D. Gilbert, J. Goldfarb and L. Herron, *Spine* **4** (1979) 78.
38.   P.S. Rae, G. Waddell and R.M. Venner, *J. Roy. Coll. Surg. Edin.* **29** (1984) 281.
39.   A.O. Ransford, D. Cairns and V. Mooney, *Spine* **1** (1976) 127.
40.   G.R. Repko and R. Cooper, *J. Clin. Psychol.* **39** (1983) 287.
41.   S.H. Roy, C.J. De Luca and D.A. Casavant, *Spine* **14** (1989) 992.
42.   S. Sacks, *Clin. Orthop.* **44** (1966) 163.
43.   R.A. Sander and J.E. Meyers, *Spine* **11** (1986) 141.
44.   J.M. Sikorski, *Spine* **10** (1985) 571.
45.   G.A. Splithoff, *J.A.M.A.* **152** (1953) 1610.
46.   R.N. Stauffer and M.B. Coventry, *J. Bone Joint Surg.* **54-A** (1972) 756.
47.   I.A.F. Stokes and J.W. Frymoyer, *Spine* **12** (1987) 688.
48.   S. Talo, N. Hendler and J. Brodie, *J. Occup. Med.* **31** (1989) 265.
49.   M.J. Tarsh and C. Royston, *Br. J. Psychiat.* **146** (1985) 18.
50.   P. Trief and N. Stein, *Arch. Phys. Med. Rehabil.* **66** (1985) 95.
51.   G. Waddell, C.J. Main, E.W. Morris, M. Di Paola and I.C.M. Gray, *Spine* **9** (1984) 209.
52.   G. Waddell, J.A. McCulloch, E. Kummel and R.M. Venner, *Spine* **5** (1980) 117.
53.   N. Wells, *London Office of Health Economics* (London 1985) 3.
54.   S.W. Wiesel, N. Tsourmas and H.L. Feffer, *Spine* **9** (1984) 549.
55.   L.L. Wiltse and P.D. Rocchio, *J. Bone Joint Surg.* **57-A** (1975) 478.
56.   W.W.K. Zung, *Arch. Gen. Psych.* **12** (1965) 63.

CHAPTER 16

FEAR-AVOIDANCE: THE NATURAL HISTORY OF BACK PAIN AND ITS MANAGEMENT

J.D.G. Troup and P.D. Slade

1. Introduction

The first experience of acute back pain can be frightening. Quite suddenly movements become guarded by the expectation of worse pain; followed by fear of its recurrence and avoidance of risk. The question is whether the fear itself may contribute to the next episode or interfere with recovery and so influence the natural course of back pain.

But the natural history of back pain is to a great extent a neglected subject, lacking a reliable science. It may not be to the fore when deciding what to do for an individual patient. And it is a subject on which clinical epidemiology has up to now produced only circumstantial evidence. The problem lies in the growing numbers of those with recurrent pain and progressive disability; in how it should be tackled. To some extent it is a clinical problem, one involving family doctors as well as hospital practice. It also offers a challenge to health education.

The tendency for symptoms of acute back pain to become chronic can not, in most cases, be explained in terms either of the morbid pathology of back pain or of the physical circumstances of its prevalence. The majority of patients with chronic symptoms have become ill because of their back pain in ways that are partly, sometimes largely, dysfunctional. It is therefore an open question whether or not therapeutic or preventive measures have been or are likely to be effective when the causes of the dysfunction remain undiagnosed and untreated: particularly if the fear is unresolved and goes unrecognised.

In the past, and still to some extent, it was believed that the origins of back and sciatic pain could be defined in specific pathological terms; and appropriate diagnostic labels attached. The logic was that back pain would, if bad enough to warrant it, be susceptible to a specific form of treatment. It was, of course, recognised that many people with back pain would get better by natural remission and that, in them, no attempt at diagnosis would be necessary. Thus the prevalence of back pain in the non-patient population was not unduly obtrusive in clinical experience. It was, indeed still is[1], widely held that nine out of ten episodes or attacks of back pain were, with or without therapy, self-limiting. Only in those with persistent or intractable pain was there a serious diagnostic problem. And so the question of a natural history did not arise. Arguments centred on diagnostic classification, based on the assorted concurrence of symptoms and clinical signs. But as they concerned diagnoses that were, at best, tentative and a group of patients the majority of whom were seldom fully, if at all, investigated; the arguments about classification were futile. In these circumstances, *"Attempting to classify back pain syndromes is like looking into a muddy fish pond.."*[2]. And so it remains.

Two things have changed. One is the growing epidemic of back trouble in commercially developed countries: with a growth rate that is out of proportion to the ætiopathology as it has been understood, implying some psychosocial phenomena in operation. And the second is the recognition that back pain has a multifactorial ætiology with many contributory factors that tend to interact. One of the factors that has to be incorporated if back pain can be said to have a natural history is the temporal component. Thus the word 'diagnosis' reverts to its original meaning: a broad understanding of the ætiognosis, of the site and origin of pain as well as the prognosis. Diagnoses can not be said to be complete, therefore, unless the early history of the complaint is known. With some prescience, an editorial in The Lancet[3] drew attention to the need to focus on the very first experience of LBT: "*The promptness and success with which the first attack of back pain is managed can therefore have a great influence on the natural course of the disease.*"

Yet in their approach to the problem of diagnosis in 1987, the Quebec Task Force on Spinal Disorders[4], though criticising the deficiencies of published research, fought shy of the concept of the natural history. Their classification of activity-related spinal disorders offered eleven categories: the first four based on symptoms, the next five being presumptive, symptom-based diagnoses, with 'chronic pain syndrome' as the tenth; followed by 'others'; all of them undefinedly 'activity-related'. The emphasis throughout was on the current attack and its course over the subsequent 4 weeks, 7 weeks and 3 months; and this has been typical of the clinical scientific approach to LBT. The 10-year study by Weber[5], comparing the results of surgical and conservative management of disc herniation, remains an exception.

The majority of patients may be taken as a group who remain largely undiagnosed. Yet they expect to be treated. They present a substantial problem in therapeutic management for health professionals. In the past, the scientist may only have been asked to identify those patients who make the least and the most demands on the service that is offered; to identify those patients who will respond poorly to a specific treatment; or to throw some light, for example, on the planning of physical therapy for patients who have to be treated anyway and the question was how best to manage the therapeutic service for them[6]. These approaches have some value in the short term but it is improbable that they would do much for the epidemic scale of LBT in the population. They beg the question of what becomes of those patients who are unlikely to respond to a standard therapeutic approach or to the type of treatment that is deemed by the auditor to be the most cost-effective. Inevitably, if the natural history of LBT in complainants is to be set aside in favour of a diagnostic label, therapy will continue to be directed at temporary relief rather than long term prevention[7].

The task of the clinical scientist is to study the natural history of low back trouble in the population and determine where and how intervention will be most effective. To begin with, a framework is needed in which to gather sets of reliable data on the total experience of LBT and its effect on the individual; on his daily activities; on the advice and treatment that have been given on each occasion; and on the outcome.

2. The multifactorial ætiology of back pain

The pain in any given patient has a multifactorial ætiology. It has stemmed from a variety of causative, contributory and interactive factors: all bearing on the biomechanical, neurophysiological and structural aspects of the pathology. And with time, more factors are added: with the responses to each treatment and with what the patient knows and understands of the variety of information and advice that has been given on each attendance. The number of variables can seem infinite: perhaps an acceptable problem for the experienced clinician but a challenge for research.

An earlier model for the multifactorial ætiology of back pain[8] depicted the interrelationships of symptoms and the related pathology and it included psychological factors. What it omitted was the temporal component: the effects of the duration of pain and disability and the cumulative effects of continued disability on the pathology. Moreover psychological factors were limited to two inputs: 'psychological stress' and 'pain-avoidance'. Now the full range of contributory, ætiological factors can perhaps be appreciated best from what are emerging as the factors that are recognised epidemiologically as predictors of back pain.

3. Predictive factors

A previous history of back trouble is one of the strongest predictive factors for further episodes. It has been widely reported. It applies to the length of the back pain history, to the number of attacks and to their duration. But there is little to go on for predicting a first attack[9-11]: just some evidence of the value of tests of physical fitness in a mainly young population. Tests of lifting strength have only been claimed to have predictive value in relation to the strength-demands at work[12,13]: not when lifting strength is tested in isolation[14].

A variety of risk indicators for back pain and its causes have been described. For back pain and sciatica they include obesity, smoking, chronic cough, psychological distress and poor general health[15]; for herniated lumbar intervertebral disc, blue-collar occupations and low or intermediate social class[16]. But it is questionable how many of these risk indicators are truly causal factors and thus improbable that many would serve as targets for therapeutic intervention in the natural history of back pain. Likewise with the study in Dayton, Ohio, which revealed that the highest prevalence of back pain was in no-longer-married women aged 50-64 years and the lowest was in educated, married men[17].

After the first attack, prediction has more scope. Injuries that are truly accidental have a worse prognosis[18-19], the trauma presumably being related to the energy input for the accident. Pain in the lower limb as well as the back leads to longer periods of absence and a greater likelihood of recurrence[20]. The clinical tests that were found to be of predictive value were described by Lloyd & Troup[18]: they include straight-leg-raising and the qualifying tests for increased root tension, the sit-up test, pain or weakness on resisted hip flexion, and back pain on passive lumbar flexion. However, these approaches to prediction rely on the effect of a single variable. It is more fruitful to study the combined effects in order to compare their predictive powers[21].

Burton & Tillotson[22] developed a multivariable model to predict the course of back trouble in 109 patients, using discriminant analysis. Prediction was determined by the combined effect of a number of variables arising from the history of back pain, from the clinical signs and other factors. The authors illustrated the relative influence of those variables that proved significant in determining whether they would show improvement or deterioration at one month after consultation: the scores for each variable having an additive effect. In a study of 1,128 patients treated in a Health Maintenance Organization in Washington, von Korff *et al.*[23] used a multivariate logistic regression analysis to predict poor outcome: the pain-grade at baseline, the duration of pain and the length of the pain-history all predicted a poor outcome.

Burton *et al.*[24] followed the progress of 252 patients given primary care for back pain after initial psychometric assessment, using a postal questionnaire 12 months later and giving a response rate of 74%. The patients were divided by their history into acute and non-acute; none of them reporting more than 52 weeks back pain and the aim was to identify predictive factors for chronicity. The number of treatments required was related to age and the duration of symptoms on presentation. Differences in the amount of psychological distress between patients with acute and non-acute pain were small but evidence of illness-behaviour was more apparent in the non-acute patients. At one year the majority of patients were better and 47% reported full recovery, allowing comparison between recovered and non-recovered groups. Using stepwise discriminant analysis 74% of all non-recovered patients could be predicted on the basis of (in the order of step entered): depression, pain-coping strategies, straight-leg-raising test, leg pain and somatic perceptions. And of the 'acute' patients with initial history of 3 weeks or less, 72% of non-recovered patients were predicted on the basis of depression, root tension signs and coping strategies. The authors concluded that psychosocial factors were dominant in the prognosis.

In the study by Burton & Tillotson[22], occupation did not emerge as a useful predictive variable. And there is growing evidence to implicate sedentary work as a risk factor[25-27]. Other occupational factors may nonetheless be significant. For example, one attempt to relate the physical work load to the risk of 'fatigue injuries' concluded with the observation that monotony, stress and job-satisfaction were more likely factors[28]. While ratings based on appraisals of employees by supervisors made six months before injury were factors reported by Bigos *et al.*[29]. Moreover, the enjoyment of work emerged as a major factor: the want of it being associated with a rate of back injury that was 2½ times greater[30]. Such occupationally related factors are not readily susceptible to intervention in the form of treatment for the individual; but as socio-ergonomic factors they may well be susceptible to intervention by management.

4. The biopsychosocial model of illness[31]

Back pain can therefore no longer be viewed in purely physical or mechanistic terms. And the dominant socioeconomic problems created by the prevalence of back trouble are centred on those in the population whose symptoms have become persistent, who have failed to respond to a variety of treatments and whose lifestyles have been adapted accordingly. For these people the focus has shifted from disease of the lower back to illness caused by their back symptoms. Of course there may have been, and still may be, an organic basis for the pain but the symptoms have become dissociated; the original injury has healed and the spine is stable; but the symptoms have persisted or become worse: diagnostically the patient has become dysfunctional. In order to assist in the recognition of this dysfunction, Waddell[31] listed a number of symptoms and signs and their interpretation: on the one hand to be regarded as normal, given the physical nature of the underlying condition; and on the other as magnified or inappropriate. Exaggerated pain-perception or illness-behaviour is a feature that is common in those with chronic back pain. But the question is how soon it can recognised or foreseen and thus either treated or prevented.

The most obvious feature in chronic back pain is avoidance-behaviour. As an epidemiological example, those in the working population who report frequent experience of back pain are notably weaker at lifting than those who have never known back pain; the former group appear to remain at or below the strength level they had achieved at the time they developed back pain, while the lifting strength of the latter group increased and reached its peak in the fourth or fifth decade[14].

5. Cognitive dimensions of chronic back pain

In those who seek treatment, much of what is learned by the patient is iatrogenic: the diagnostic label, the need for pain-killers and subsequent medication and the prescription of rest. And to that mixture, add the knowledge that on return to work, the symptoms have not disappeared; medication is still taken, but with little conviction that it does any good. Alternatively, that there may be no job to return to. Much else comes from experience and the quest for the relief of pain. Symptoms are exaggerated in the hope of persuading the clinician to investigate further or try some other treatment. And, secondarily, depression and anxiety become manifest: symptoms which are not infrequently treated symptomatically with further medication. Not surprisingly, learned helplessness becomes a major cognitive feature[32].

Symonds *et al.*[33] conducted a survey of 466 workers in a multi-task-factory using 'back-beliefs' and 'psychosocial aspects of work' questionnaires: workers were grouped to compare those who had reported more than one week of absence due to back trouble with those with less or no such absence; absence being associated with external locus of control and negative beliefs about back pain. In other words, a basis for learned helplessness.

6. Fear-avoidance

Underlying much of the illness-behaviour in patients with chronic back pain is fear. Fear of pain that may recur and fear of the unknown, perhaps of some unrecognised and serious disease. In their Fear-Avoidance Model of Exaggerated Pain-Perception, Lethem *et al.*[34] showed how the fear originates from injury or the experience of acute back pain. The model then showed how the fear could on the one hand be contained or confronted, in which case the individual would progress to full recovery and rehabilitation; or, on the other hand, how the fear stays unrelieved, leading to persistent symptoms, exaggerated pain-perception and avoidance. Just which route the patient takes depends on the psychosocial dynamic in which the disability operates, on individual personality as well as iatrogenic factors and thus on how the individual has learned to cope with pain[35].

Fear-avoidance was assessed by a questionnaire on pain history and its severity; on pain-coping-strategies; personality and previous life-events. Using this model, Rose *et al.*[36] compared the results in patients with chronic back pain, post-herpetic neuralgia and reflex sympathetic dystrophy with those in recovered groups and demonstrated that fear-avoidance was not peculiar to people with back pain; that the model *"..provides a unified psychological theory which explains the development of chronic pain resulting from a benign, acute pain experience.."*. Waddell *et al.*[37] developed a Fear-Avoidance Beliefs Questionnaire with high reproducibility and showed that fear-avoidance beliefs about back pain and work accounted for a substantial proportion of disability, independent of the severity of pain itself.

In order to test the hypothesis that exaggerated pain-behaviour, particularly fear-avoidance, in patients with back pain was not solely a feature of the chronicity of their pain, Klenerman *et al.*[38] studied patients presenting with acute low back pain in general practice. They showed that fear-avoidance variables were the most successful in predicting outcome. They concluded that fear of pain was recognisable at the earliest stage of the experience of back pain; and that it should arguably be included in the therapeutic approach during the acute phase of back pain.

Fear-avoidance should therefore be seen as part of the ætiological picture of back pain, acute or chronic. If the fear goes unrecognised and untreated, the risk is not merely failure to recover but adaptation to non-use and the added risk of accelerated degeneration[39].

7. Intervention in the natural history of back pain

The need for early and active treatment of acute back pain has gained recognition and likewise the need to limit the duration of bed-rest[40]. At the same time a number of rehabilitation programmes have been developed for the management of chronically disabled, dysfunctional patients[23,41-43]. Their successes are not wholly comparable as they have detailed differences in the types of patients who attend and differences in the methods of their referral; as well as differences in psychometric assessment and the types of psychotherapy on offer. Some of the programmes pay attention to the relief of fear though not as a specific aim of treatment.

Reilly[32] describes a pain management programme in Liverpool for 42 patients with chronic low back pain who were referred from general practice and from an orthopædic clinic. The programme was managed by a graduate psychologist and a research physiotherapist. And the significant difference from other therapeutic programmes for such patients is that other management features such as medication and certification of fitness for work, remained under the control of their referring clinician. This is quite distinct from the absolute control of therapy exercised in many of the programmes in the USA. Moreover there was no control or influence on return to work as the programme took place in a region of high unemployment. The programme lasted 5 days and totalled 18 hours: it included cognitive therapy, target-setting, relaxation therapy and exercise therapy. The patients acted as their own controls because their symptoms remained unchanged between the time of initial assessment and the start of the course: 10-12 weeks. Six months later both pain ratings and medication remained unchanged. But psychometric assessments showed improvements in depression, in the ability to control pain, in self-belief and in responsibility and thus benefits in the form of helplessness unlearned.

Reilly[32] had postulated that group-treatment would have advantages over individual treatment: therefore 22 patients were treated in groups and 20 individually. There were few differences in outcome. But the results indicated that individual therapy may have some advantages in enhancing physical fitness and reducing functional disability. And the probability is that the advantages or disadvantages of group or individual therapy will vary from one patient to the next. Though the economies of group-therapy are obvious the points at which some patients merit individual attention have yet to be defined. Further research is in progress and subsequent work by Reilly and his colleagues indicates that refresher courses in pain management will have their place.

8. Conclusions

The prevalence of back trouble in the population, the tendency of acute back pain to recur and the epidemic increase in those with chronic disability is evidence that little is to be gained by focussing epidemiologically or therapeutically on isolated episodes of pain. The duty to eliminate serious underlying disease, of course, remains. And in those who fail to make a full recovery and whose disability is progressive investigation with a view to surgery is the logical step. In a small proportion surgery may be justified but that leaves the great majority for whom it can not.

The natural history of the progression to chronicity from the first experience of back pain is bound up with the biopsychosocial model of illness-behaviour of which fear-avoidance is a dominant factor. But it is now evident that illness-behaviour and pain-avoidance are susceptible to treatment to alleviate the fear of pain, the fear of the future, and the learned helplessness and depression which are features of chronicity. It is now possible and fruitful to intervene therapeutically in the natural history of back pain and bring it under control; and that the most suitable time for intervention is during primary care. The question though is how this can be planned.

The pain management programmes that are cited above all relied on the participation of clinical psychologists: on professional skills that are not widely available and certainly not enough to staff all centres of primary care. Yet patients with back pain are economically the most demanding of those with musculoskeletal disorders and there are clear benefits if their numbers are to be stemmed and reduced. The challenge lies partly with those responsible for primary care in family, occupational health and hospital practice; but also in the field of health education.

9. References

1. American Academy of Orthopaedic Surgeons, in *Knowledge update 3: home study syllabus* (Park Ridge, Illinois: American Academy of Orthopaedic Surgeons).
2. R.W. Porter, in *Back pain: classification of back syndromes*, ed. J.C.T. Fairbank and & P.B. Pynsent (Manchester University Press: Manchester) p. 117.
3. The Lancet (editorial), *Lancet* **2** (1984) 1020.
4. Quebec Task Force on Spinal Disorders, *Spine* **12** (1987) S1.
5. H. Weber, *Spine* **8** (1983) 131.
6. C.E. Coxhead, H. Inskip, T.W. Meade, W.R.S. North and J.D.G. Troup, *Lancet* **1** (1981) 1065.
7. H. Weber and A.K. Burton, *Clinical Biomechanics* **1** (1986) 160.
8. J.D.G. Troup, *Scand. J. Work Environ. Health* **10** (1984) 419.
9. B. Nordgren, R. Schelé and K. Linroth, *Scand J. Rehabil. Med.* **12** (1980) 1.
10. M.J. Karvonen, J.T. Viitasalo, P.V. Komi, J. Nummi and T. Järvinen, *Scand J. Rehabil. Med.* **12** (1980) 53.
11. F. Biering-Sórensen, *Spine* **9** (1984) 106.
12. D.B. Chaffin, G.D. Herrin and W.M. Keyserling, *J. Occup. Med.* **20** (1978) 403
13. W.M. Keyserling, G.D. Herrin and D.B. Chaffin, *J. Occup. Med.* **22** (1980) 332.
14. J.D.G. Troup, T.K. Foreman, C.E. Baxter and D. Brown, *Spine* **12** (1987) 645.
15. M. Heliövaara, *Ann. Med.* **21** (1989) 257.
16. M. Heliövaara, P. Knekt and A. Aromaa, *J. Chron. Dis.* **40** (1987) 251.
17. L.S. Reisbord and S. Greenland, *J. Chron. Dis.* **38** (1985) 691.
18. D.C.E.F. Lloyd and J.D.G. Troup, *J. Soc. Occup. Med.* **33** (1983) 66.
19. S.J. Bigos, D.M. Spengler, N.A. Martin, J. Zeh, L. Fisher, A. Nachemson and M.H. Wang, *Spine* **11** (1986) 246.
20. G.B.J. Andersson, *Spine* **6** (1981) 53.
21. A.K. Burton, K.M. Tillotson and J.D.G. Troup, *Spine* **14** (1989) 939.
22. A.K. Burton and K.M. Tillotson, *Spine* **16** (1991) 7.
23. M. von Korff, R.A. Deyo, D. Cherkin and W. Barlow, *Spine* **18** (1993) 855.
24. A.K. Burton, K.M. Tillotson, C.J. Main and S. Hollis, *Spine* **20** (1995) in press.
25. H. Riihimäki, S. Tola, T. Videman and K. Hänninen, *Spine* **14** (1989) 204.

26. H. Riihimäki, E. Viikari-Juntura, G. Moneta, J. Kuha, T. Videman and S. Tola, *Spine* **19** (1994) 138.
27. T. Videman, M. Nurminen and J.D.G. Troup, *Spine* **15** (1990) 728.
28. M. Magnusson, M. Grandqvist, R. Jonson, V. Lindell, U. Lundberg, L. Wallin and T. Hansson, *Spine* **15** (1990) 774.
29. S.J. Bigos, D.M. Spengler, N.A. Martin, J. Zeh, L. Fisher and A. Nachemson, *Spine* **11** (1986) 252.
30. S.J. Bigos, M.C. Battié, D.M. Spengler, L.D. Fisher, W.E. Fordyce, T.H. Hansson, A.L. Nachemson and M.D. Wortley, *Spine 16 (1991) 1.*
31. G. Waddell, *Spine* **12** (1987) 632.
32. J.P. Reilly, *PhD Thesis*, University of Liverpool.
33. T.L. Symonds, A.K. Burton, K.M. Tillotson and C.J. Main, *Spine* **20** (1995) in press.
34. J. Lethem, P.D. Slade, J.D.G. Troup and G. Bentley, *Behav. Res. Therapy* **21** (1983) 401.
35. P.D. Slade, J.D.G. Troup, J. Lethem and G. Bentley, *Behav. Res. Therapy* **21** (1983) 409.
36. M.J. Rose, L. Klenerman, L. Aitchison and P. D. Slade, *Behav. Res. Therapy* **30** (1992) 359.
37. G. Waddell, M. Newton, I. Henderson, D. Somerville and C.J. Main, *Pain* **52** (1993) 157.
38. L. Klenerman, P.D. Slade, I.M. Stanley, B. Pennie, M.J. Rose, J. P. Reilly, L.E. Aitchison and J.D.G. Troup, *Spine* **20** (1995) in press.
39. J.D.G . Troup and T. Videman, *Clin. Biomechanics* **4** (1989) 173.
40. R.A. Deyo, A.K. Diehl and M. Rosenthal, *New Engl. J. Med.* **315** (1986) 1064.
41. T.G. Mayer, R.J. Gatchel, N. Kishono, J. Keeley, P. Capra, H. Mayer, J. Barnett and V. Mooney, *Spine* **10** (1985) 482.
42. C.J. Main and H. Parker, in *Back pain: new approaches to rehabilitation and education*, ed. M. Roland and J. Jenner (Manchester: Manchester University Press) p. 128.
43. R.G. Hazard, J.W. Fenwick, S.M. Kalisch, J. Redmond, V. Reeves, S. Ried and J.W. Frymoyer, *Spine* **14** (1989) 157.
44. G. Mellin, K. Härkäpää, H. Vanharanta, M. Hupli, R. Heinonen and A. Järvikoski, *Spine* **18** (1993) 825.
45. M.W. Werneke, D.E. Harris and R.L. Lichter, *Spine* **18** (1993) 2412.
46. H. Alaranta, U. Rytökoski, A. Rissanen, S. Talo, T. Rönnemaa, P. Puukka, S-L. Karppi, T. Videman, V. Kallio and P. Slätis, *Spine* **19** (1994) 1339.

CHAPTER 17

CHEMONUCLEOLYSIS

M. Sullivan

1. Introduction

Chymopapain has had a very dificult history over the last thirty years. It is probably the most investigated drug and still remains controversial. During the sixties and seventies it became increasingly more popular in North America but also there were more and more complications because it was being used by untrained physicians. Then, in 1976, Schwetsenau[1], at the Walter Reid Hospital, did a double blind study and showed that the enzyme was ineffectual. The study was flawed completely for a number of reasons, the most important being that a chelating agent had been used in the trial. A second double blind study was done by Fraser in 1982[2] in which he found completely different results in that the enzyme was effective and considerably better than placebo. A number of subsequent blind studies have been done, all of which have confirmed this. Because of the fact that all discs tend to resolve, any placebo effect will have a cure rate. Henrik Weber in 1983[3] showed that discs resolve without any treatment.

The ideal patient for chemonucleolysis is under the age of forty and has profound back and leg pain, with more leg than back. Straight leg raising should be limited on the affected side and the patient may or may not have cross leg pain. There should be a neurological deficit - either motor, sensory or reflex - and a neuro-radiographic investigation should correlate with the clinical signs. It is felt that a CT scan is an inadequate investigation unless combined with myelography. Myelography on its own is acceptable but the investigation of choice is Magnetic Resonance Imaging. Other investigations should be undertaken. Plain radiographs should be normal, as should routine blood tests. These patients, of course, are the ideal ones for surgery as well as for chemonucleolysis. They should have adequate conservative treatment, which should include a week in bed. There is no evidence that more than one week's bed rest is of any value. A further two to three weeks of analgesics and physiotherapy should be undertaken unless there is a cauda equina lesion. One should neither inject nor operate on a disc in under three weeks from the date of onset.

The procedure can be undertaken either in the operating theatre or the radiology department. There must be two dimensional image intensification to make sure the needle is placed exactly in the centre of the disc. Many of the severe complications have been caused by using inadequate image intensification. There are certain contra-indications: as the enzyme is a foreign protein there is a 1 in 150 chance of acute anaphylaxis in North America but 1 in 700 in Europe. The difference could be in the use of papain - used commercially as a meat tenderiser and also as a contact lens cleaner. These two facilities are not used as commonly in Europe as in North America. An absolute contra-indication has been re-injection but Deutman[4] does not agree. Should patients have an anaphylactic reaction, large doses of adrenalin are needed and so one should not inject patients with cardiac problems. It may seem that an acute disc prolapse in a patient who has had a recent myocardial infarct would be ideally treated with chymopapain but this is not so and should not be done. Also, the enzyme should not be used during pregnancy and is, of course, unsuitable if there is any evidence of spinal stenosis. In our view this should not be undertaken at the extremes of age - Sullivan 1992[5]. In the young adolescent disc it is more usual for the end plate to separate and therefore simply decompressing the nucleus will not relieve the symptoms. In the elderly the disc contains very little proteoglycan and consists almost entirely of collagen. However, as Benoist *et al.*[6] have shown, chemonucleolysis can be a very effective treatment in the elderly.

If one is going to treat a disc prolapse by minimal invasion therapy there are basically three options - discolysis with chymopapain, percutaneous disc removal (either manual or automated) and laser discectomy. In all three the discs should be contained or, in the case of chymopapain, it can also be sub-ligamentous. None of these modalities are effective for a sequestrated fragment. It is often extremely difficult to diagnose a sequestrated fragment clinically. High definition MRI will often show the fragment but this investigation is not always available and even when it is, it is not infallible. One of the more common reasons for failure of minimal invasion therapy is a sequestrated fragment which needs to be removed surgically.

Which of these three modalities to use? We would suggest always using chymopapain at the L5/S1 level as, to get a rigid wide bore instrument into the 5/1 space, without damaging the sacral end plate is always very difficult and not infrequently impossible. This is particularly true of laser discectomy with the end plate is burned. With chemonucleolysis one can bend the needle to enter the lumbo-sacral space. At levels above L4 any of these three modalities is acceptable and the results of all three methods are almost identical, with about 75% success at one year. However, chymopapain is considerably cheaper. The cost of the Holmium YAG laser that is now used is £120,000. When the enzyme was first used it was thought that high doses of five thousand units per disc space were essential. We now know that two thousand units per disc is quite adequate which has both eased the cost and lessened the amount of back ache.

2. Results

During the period 1973 to 1988 we injected 412 patients at the Royal National Orthopaedic Hospital. In that same period 2,000 backs were operated upon. Only about 20% of patients with root pain are suitable for chemonucleolysis. Of these 412 patients, 60 were treated during 1973/74. Many of them were unsuitable in that they had had previous surgery or had psychological problems.

The results were poor. By 1975 the the patient selection criteria had improved. From 1975 to 1978, 90 patients were treated with chemonucleolysis and these have now been followed up for ten years[7]. In this group there was a 75% success rate at one year and the same at ten years, although they were not exactly the same patients. No series has shown a 75% success rate at ten years following routine surgery. Our results are very similar to those of other observers around the world.

3. Complications and safety

In our 412 patients the complications rates were:

Cauda equina lesion	0
Paraplegia	0
Disc infection	2
Persistent severe back pain	12
Acute anaphylaxis	0
Giant Hives	1
Subsequent surgery	23

The infected disc spaces did not produce organisms but showed disc space narrowing and end-plate erosion. These settled with antibiotics and time.

In 1976, six surgeons were using this technique in Europe. By 1989 there were 316 surgeons and they had treated 44,000 patients. By far the biggest users were France and Germany. Out of these patients there were 61 cases of anaphylaxis (1.4 per thousand)[8]. These were treated correctly and there were no deaths or subsequent sequelae. This is in marked contrast to North America. The disc infection rate was 2.5 per thousand (102). These were all treated conservatively and no-one needed anterior fusion. There were 3 serious complications - one meningeal haemorrhage and two cases of paraplegia when the drug was injected intrathecally. The single most worrying post operative complication was back pain, of which there were 1,202 or 28 per thousand. Since the introduction of Bupivacaine this has now dropped to less than 1%.

4. Summary

Chemonucleolysis is an excellent treatment for the patient with a contained disc prolapse, giving a 75% success rate at ten years. This is better than any surgical series.

5. References

1.   P. R. Schwetsenau, A. Ramirez, J. Johnson *et al*, *J Neurosurgery* **45** (1976) 622.
2.   R. D. Fraser, *Spine* **7** (1982) 608.
3.   H. Weber, *Spine* **8** (1983) 131-140.
4.   R. Deutman, *Orthopaedics* **1 4** (1993) 333-339.
5.   M. Sullivan, *Surgery of the Spine*, ed. Findlay and Owen (1992) 733-736.
6.   M. Benoist, H. Parent, M. Nisard, B. Lassale, A. Deburge, *Revue du Rhumatisme* **60(6)** (1994) 435-439.
7.   M. Sullivan, M, Results of chymopapain and discography. Presented at International Intradiscal Therapy Society, March 1989, Orlando, Florida.
8.   R. Bouillet, *Acta. Orthop. Belg.* **49** (1983) 48.

CHAPTER 18

EXPERIENCE WITH CHEMONUCLEOLYSIS

D. Wardlaw

1. Introduction

Chemonucleolysis as a treatment for sciatica due to soft disc herniation has now been used for more than 30 years. It was introduced by Lyman Smith in 1961 and is now widely used in North America, Europe and Australasia. The world literature on the subject is vast and consistently supports the use of Chymopapain. Chemonucleolysis, and the procedure has now withstood the test of time. My own first hand experience of the technique commenced in 1981 where I had the opportunity of learning to perform the technique under the excellent tuition of Dr John McCulloch, then of St Michael's Hospital in Toronto. I subsequently introduced it into Grampian by carrying out a prospective randomised study with review by an independent observer, Dr Clifford Eastmond, Consultant Rheumatologist, City Hospital, Aberdeen, and this confirmed its value. I have performed further studies which have confirmed the efficacy of chemonucleolysis, and in my own mind they have helped me develop a very clear understanding of the technique. These articles are discussed together with a review of the world literature in an article entitled "The Case for Chemonucleolysis"[1].

Chymopapain was first isolated from the latex of the papaya plant by Jansen and Balls in 1941[2]. Its potential in the management of intervertebral disc disease was first recognised by Lyman Smith in 1959, then an orthopaedic surgeon in Illinois, USA when he happened to read the article. He subsequently tested the potential of Chymopapain chemonucleolysis by injection of intervertebral discs in animals. He published these findings in the first article on the subject of Chymopapain chemonucleolysis in Nature in 1963[3]. One year later he published the first article entitled "The Enzyme Dissolution of the Nucleus Pulposus in Humans"[4]. Subsequently larger series were published by himself and over the subsequent years by many other authors[5-10].

Despite the fact that Smith clearly recognised the clinical indications and the potential of the procedure for the treatment of sciatica, it was perceived by many surgeons as a 'cure-all' for patients with back pain problems, and because it was an injection technique, it was seen as a lesser procedure. The potential risks were not properly appreciated by those who took it up. There were no restrictions on who could perform the procedure and there was no requirement for formal training. As a result in the early 1970's many problems and complications arose which should never have occurred. The perception of the procedure at that time is, in my opinion encapsulated in the first double-blind study which was carried out in the United States and concluded that chemonucleolysis did not have a significantly better success rate compared to a placebo[11,12]. There were many criticisms over this trial, but in my opinion the most relevant one was poor patient selection! Nevertheless as a result of this trial, F.D.A. approval for the procedure was withdrawn in the United States. The medico-legal climate in the United States meant that even when the procedure was given approval again in 1982, it was impossible for many surgeons to offer it to their patients, because of the bad publicity and the medicolegal climate. There were also political reasons for what happened in a country which compared to the U.K. has up to ten times the number of surgeons per head of the population, from two competing specialties offering treatment to patients. Meanwhile, Britain as always tended to follow the United States in that the procedure was not popular. However, it was widely practised on the continent of Europe, particularly France, Belgium, Holland and Germany.

In 1982, an excellent double-blind study was published by Rob Fraser from Adelaide, Australia clearly demonstrating a success rate for chemonucleolysis of 80% compared to a placebo success of 57% at one year[13]. Three year follow-up subsequently demonstrated a success rate of 73% and 47% respectively[14]. The publication of Fraser's study allowed Javid in the United States under the auspices of the FDA to perform a further double blind study in 108 patients. This demonstrated a chemonucleolysis success rate of 73% compared to a placebo success of 42%[15]. Following this trial the drug was once again licensed in the United States and the results were confirmed by further studies.

Retrospective studies have shown a long term success rate of 76% for a 9-20 year follow-up and 85% long term follow-up at 1-10 years has been demonstrated compared to 80.3% success rate in a comparable surgical group of patients[16-25]. The long term efficacy of chemonucleolysis was finally confirmed by a ten year follow-up of Fraser's initial study clearly demonstrating a chemonucleolysis success rate of 80% compared to a placebo success of 34%[26]. Clearly the value of chemonucleolysis as an interventional treatment for patients suffering from the effects of sciatica was demonstrated to be very significantly better than placebo treatment or to treatment by physiotherapy or simply 'doing nothing' as suggested by Weber[27]

2. Personal experience

My own experience with chemonucleolysis started in my reading of the literature as a Senior Registrar in the late 1970's. In 1981 I was lucky enough to have the opportunity to visit Toronto on a six month leave of absence from my consultant post. I worked primarily alongside Professor Ian Macnab of the Wellesley Hospital and luckily had the opportunity to visit and learn from the many world-renowned spinal surgeons who were then working in the city. One of them was Dr John McCulloch whom I was very keen to visit because of the interest I had already developed in the technique of chemonucleolysis. Ian Macnab, a long-time friend of Lyman Smith, had been an early pioneer in the use of chemonucleolysis. Under his auspices the technique was evaluated in Toronto and taken up by many surgeons in Canada and particularly by John McCulloch who became world famous for his work in the field. I was introduced to the procedure and very quickly allowed, under John's supervision, to carry out the procedure on many patients. At that time, the majority of patients referred to Toronto for chemonucleolysis were from the United States where the procedure was not available. Patients were referred to surgeons in Canada and many of them flew into Toronto for an out-patient consultation and if they were diagnosed as suitable for chemonucleolysis the procedure was performed the following day as a day case. They then left hospital to stay for one or two nights in a local hotel or with relatives before flying back home. Thousands of patients received treatment in this way.

I was convinced of the value of the technique but concerned by the scepticism of colleagues, locally and in the UK. In 1982, therefore, I set up a prospective randomised study of chemonucleolysis compared to surgery for the management of sciatica for soft disc herniation.

3. Prospective randomised study of chemonucleolysis versus surgery for soft disc herniation in 100 cases[28]

3.1. Material and methods

All patients entered into this particular study had the typical symptoms and signs of sciatica as described by McCulloch and MacNab[29], and whose symptoms had failed to respond to three months of conservative management including two weeks hospital bed rest with or without traction. All patients had at least dominant leg pain, reduced straight leg raising, and a positive water soluble myelogram. I personally carried out the treatment in all patients and independent follow-up was carried out by Dr Clifford Eastmond, now Consultant Rheumatologist, Aberdeen Royal Infirmary. Patients were followed-up post-injection or surgery at six weeks, three months, six months and one year and assessed for persistence of back or leg pain, time of return to work or normal activities and as to whether they were completely better, significantly improved, the same or worse. During the course of this study I had operating lists in three different hospitals and so from the organisational point of view, the collection of data had to be minimised.

100 patients were entered into the study by computer randomisation according to age (less than 40 years and 40 years and over), sex (male or female) and level (L5/S1, L4/5 and above L4/5).

If patients suited the above criteria they were offered treatment either by surgery, the standard treatment at the time or by chemonucleolysis which was described as involving the chemical digestion as opposed to the surgical removal of the 'soft centre' and protruding portion of the disc. Patients were advised that if they entered the study then neither they nor myself would decide the treatment which was by a computer randomisation. An initial description of a soft disc herniation causing root entrapment was given to the patient to ensure a simple understanding of the problem in relation to treatments offered. Patients were advised that chemonucleolysis was likely to be slightly less effective than surgery and that if no relief was obtained by six weeks post-injection then surgery would be offered.

3.2 Technique of chemonucleolysis

Chemonucleolysis was carried out by placing the patient in the left lateral position with a small pad if necessary under the waist to straighten the lumbar spine (Figure 1), using the Lateral Approach (see below). X-ray image intensifier was used to control needle position in the antero-posterior (AP) and lateral views. Ten millilitres of 1% Lignocaine are injected to skin and muscle down the needle track.

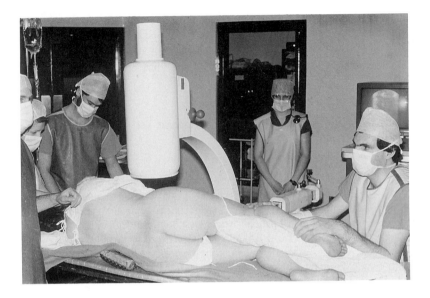

Figure 1. Patient in the left lateral position to straighten the lumbar spine.

The needle entry position is just above the iliac crest for the L4/5 and L5/S1 discs and just over one hands breadth from the mid line in the average-sized patient (Figure 2). In larger patients a more lateral entry point is required. For this entry point the needle passes at an angle between 45-60° from the horizontal; and pointing almost directly medially towards the L4/5 disc, or caudally 20-30° in a medial direction for the L5/S1 disc. A 4" 18 gauge needle was inserted down to the annulus of the disc (Figure 3) and a straight or curved 22 gauge needle was inserted through it into the centre of the nucleus pulposus. Check X-rays were taken to ensure accurate needle placement in the centre of the disc in the AP (Figure 4(a)) and lateral (Figure 4(b)) views. The level was carefully correlated with the patient's symptoms and affected level on myelography. It was felt essential not to risk either potentially altering the action of Chymopapain (Discase) or increasing the risk of complications by discography or discometry. Discase, 8 mg in 2 ml sterile water was slowly injected into the disc and an airstrip dressing applied over the skin puncture. Chymodiactin is the preparation now used. Prior to injection 0.5 ml neopam is injected to exclude the tiny proportion of intradural protrusions which occur.
    The full instrumentation for the procedure is as follows;
            Warmed Betadine for skin preparation
            1 x 10 ml syringe for injection of 10 ml 1% Lignocaine with one small and
            one larger needle.
            1 x filling cannula
            1 x 18 gauge x 4" or 5" needle

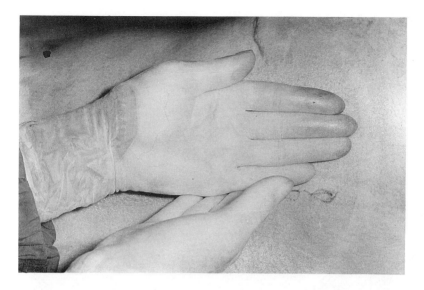

Figure 2. Needle entry is one-hands breadth from the midline in the average patient.

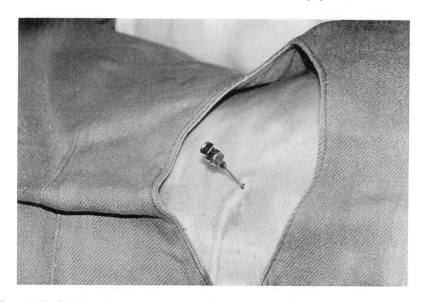

Figure 3. Needle inserted into the centre of the disc

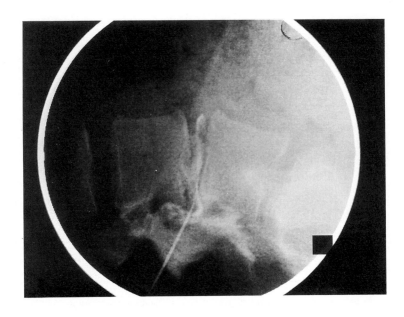

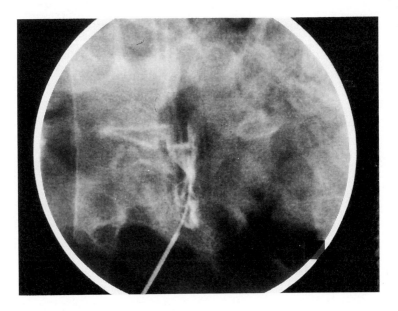

Figure 4. (a) Antero-posterior and (b) lateral x-rays to ensure that the needle is placed in the centre of the disc.

1 x 22 gauge x 7" needle
1 x 5 ml syringe with filling needle
1 injection tube to carry out discogram
1 x 2 ml syringe for chymopapain injection
1 Airstrip dressing.

3.3. The lateral approach to the disc[30]

The posterior (Figure 5 position A) and postero-lateral (Figure 5 position B) approach to the disc used by many surgeons in the past traverse the spinal canal and carries serious risks. The posterior approach in fact always goes transdurally whilst the postero-lateral approach may in many instances actually miss the dura but there is serious risk of causing dural or neural damage. The only safe approach is the lateral approach (Figure 5 position C) in which the needle is passed percutaneously just over one hand's breadth from the midline; the actual distance varying depending on the external circumference of the patient (Figure 5). The ideal position to penetrate the disc is on the postero-lateral corner (Figure 6). At this point the exiting nerve root passes superior to the disc (Figure 7) and if the disc is entered at this point the needle will invariably reach a point close to the centre of the nucleus pulposus. The author prefers the two needle technique in which an 18 gauge 4" or 5" needle is passed down to the annulus of the disc and a smaller 22 gauge 7" needle is railroaded through this and then passed through the annulus into the nucleus. A 22 gauge needle can be curved so that as it exits from the 18 gauge needle it curves as it traverses the tissues and thereby can in fact 'turn corners'.

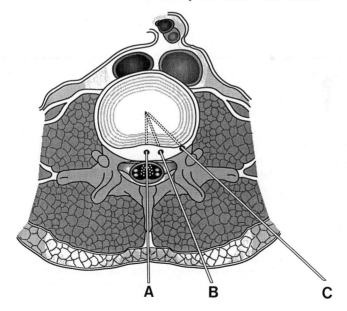

A   B   C

Figure 5. Posterior (A), postero-lateral (B) and lateral (C) approaches to the disc.

3.4. Technique of anaesthesia for chemonucleolysis

All patients were given initially a pre-medication of Omnopon 15-20 mg and Scopolamine, 0.3-0.4 mg with pre-operative Diazepam in first cases and laterally with Medazolam (Hypnovel), 5-10 mg titrated as necessary. Approximately 10 cm^3 of 1% Lignocaine was injected into skin and muscle down the needle track prior to insertion of the needle. Initially this was given without additional anaesthesia, but it was found that the injection was very often painful and therefore intravenous Methohexiton sodium (Brietal) 1 mg/kg was given intravenously prior to the injection. Propofol (Diprevan) is now preferred to Brietal. These drugs ensure a still patient during the injection with rapid recovery of consciousness and amnesia for the procedure in almost all patients.

3.5. Surgical technique

Surgery was carried out with the patient under general anaesthesia in the kneeling position. A small midline incision was made retracting the paraspinal muscles laterally from the midline of the affected side. The appropriate amount of bone was removed from the adjacent laminae and facets, the ligamentum flavum removed, the root and dura retracted medially, the disc protrusion incised and disc enucleation carried out. A free fat graft was applied over the defect and a suction drain inserted before wound closure. Post-operatively patients treated by chemonucleolysis were allowed home after one or two days. Rarely, they were kept in hospital for a day or two longer, either due to fairly severe low back pain or unrelieved leg pain. Surgery patients were kept in hospital usually for about a week. Occasionally they were allowed home a day or two earlier and on one occasion hospitalisation was required for three weeks.

3.6. Post-procedural advice to patients

Patients treated by both methods were given the same post-operative advice. They were advised to take it very easy for the first week, resting lying down, not sitting and to sit only for meals. They were to gradually get up slowly for short walks as tolerated and they were all given an advice sheet. In general they were advised not to return to light work for four to six weeks, moderately heavy work for three months and very heavy work for six months. The reason for this was that we were basically carrying out similar procedures on the disc, in one case the chemical digestion of the nucleus pulposus and the protrusion[31-33] and in the other the surgical removal and as far as mobilisation was concerned there was no back treatment bias.

3.7. Failure of chemonucleolysis

Chemonucleolysis was deemed to have failed if the patient was no better as six weeks post-injection when surgery was offered and was carried out at the earliest opportunity.

3.8. Radiological parameters[34]

Disc height as an estimate of disc degeneration was measured by comparing the affected disc to an adjacent normal disc expressed as a percentage. The method of assessment was tested on normal spine and was found to be accurate.

The myelogram size was classified according to the Postacchini method[35].

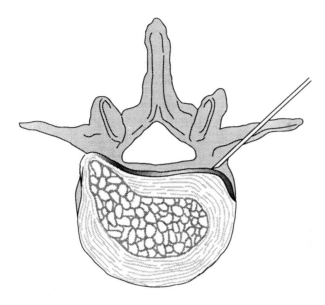

Figure 6. Correct placement of needle for entry to the nucleus.

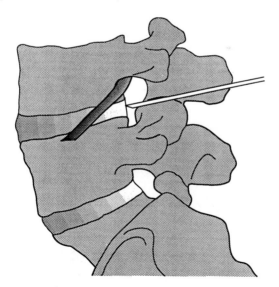

Figure 7. Needle tip on the posterior border of the vertebral body; the nerves pass superior to the disc.

3.9. Results

The randomisation resulted in a group of 100 patients in whom 98 had disc protrusions at either the L4/5 level (second last mobile level, SLML) and the L5/S1 level (the last mobile level, LML) and two protrusions occurred at L3/4 level. 48 patients were treated by chemonucleolysis of whom 27 were males, one of whom had a protrusion at L3/4 level, 13 at the SLML and 13 at the LML. There were 21 females with nine protrusions at the SLML and 12 at the LML. 52 patients had surgery of whom 33 were male, one protrusion occurring at L3/4, 19 at SLML and 13 at LML. There were 19 female patients with 10 protrusions at SLML. These findings are comparable to other unselected series.

In total there were 40 female patients of whom 18 were aged under 40 and 22 were aged 40 or more. There were 60 male patients, 33 under 40 and 27 aged 40 or more. The age range in the whole series was 18-64 years.

The chemonucleolysis procedure took on average one-third of the theatre time (25 minutes) compared to disc enucleation (1 hour 15 minutes) and this included the total theatre time including the time taken for induction of anaesthesia and recovery in theatre. The average hospital stay for chemonucleolysis patients averaged four days compared to eight days following disc enucleation. In general chemonucleolysis patients were allowed home on the second post-operative day. Very occasionally due to unrelieved leg pain or acute back pain, they were kept in hospital for longer. Post-surgery patients were generally kept in hospital for about a week and occasionally were allowed home earlier. One patient required hospitalisation for just over three weeks post-surgery, having developed severe wound infection (see under Complications).

10 of the 48 patients treated by chemonucleolysis did not respond to treatment and required surgery. The findings were compared to the 52 patients treated primarily by surgery. This suggested that the majority of extruded discs and half-sequestrated disc had responded to chemonucleolysis. Eight of these patients responded to surgery.

3.10. Complications

One patient had a very large protrusion causing virtually complete block on myelogram and post-injection developed a cauda equina syndrome. She was treated by immediate exploration and a large extruded disc was removed. Functionally she had an excellent result but due to the fact that she still had very slight diffuse sensory disturbance in the L5/S1 dermatomes she was classified as improved. She had no bladder or bowel symptoms. In retrospect she subsequently admitted to a history of urinary hesitancy prior to injection.

One surgical patient at operation had a small dural tear. This was repaired. Post-operatively all was well and she was covered with prophylactic antibiotic in the form of Penicillin and Sulphadimidine. In spite of this she developed a spreading cellulitis in both loins in conjunction with some neurological disturbance in her lower leg. The infection proved to be due to a hospital resistant staphylococcus and this ultimately responded to treatment, but unfortunately she was left with a diffuse Grade 3/4 weakness with some bladder and bowel disturbance and some diffuse sensory loss in her lower limbs and trunk secondary to staphylococcal meningitis.

3.11. Radiological analysis

The greatest degree of disc degeneration showed disc height of 20% and indeed overall 34 patients had disc height 20-60%, 33 - 61-80% and 33 - 81-100%. The degree of disc degeneration was evenly spread throughout males and females and throughout those patients treated by chemonucleolysis and surgery. It was also spread evenly throughout the age groups which suggests that degenerative disc disease is not directly a function of age, but rather a function of a disease process.

There was no relationship found between the duration of back pain or leg pain history versus disc height. The size of the myelographic defect broken into small, medium and large groups were fairly evenly spread between surgery and chemonucleolysis. There was no relationship of the size of myelographic defect to duration of back pain or leg pain or to response to Chemonucleolysis or surgery.

Of the 10 chemonucleolysis failures, eight of them were under 40 years of age and two of them were over 40. There was no difference in the overall success rate of those patients treated by chemonucleolysis compared to the surgical group and indeed breaking to two groups into those aged over 40 and those aged under 40 showed no statistical difference between any of the groups. There were no patients who remained the same or worse and were aged 40 or over. The only finding of statistical significance was that those patients with a history of six months or less had a success rate of 86.2% due to the chemonucleolysis alone compared to those with a history of more that six months who had a success rate of 56.3% (P=0.035).

3.12. Conclusions

The overall conclusions of the study confirmed by other authors were that chemonucleolysis was successful in 79% of cases and 80% of failures responded to subsequent surgery such that the overall results are at least as good as those patients treated primarily by surgery[35-41]. Spinal surgery is therefore unnecessary in 79% of cases. Time in hospital is half of that compared to surgery on average and theatre time is one-third. The procedure is safe and easier for the patient and surgeon. Pre-injection disc height or disc degeneration is unrelated to age or outcome and age itself is unrelated to eventual outcome although the majority of chemonucleolysis failures were in the lower age group. The size of the myelographic defect is unrelated to the surgical finding or outcome although Postacchini who studied a larger series of patients suggested that for large herniations with severe symptoms surgery is preferred. Six of seven extruded segments and half the sequestrated discs appeared to respond to chemonucleolysis. A history of back pain of any duration is unrelated to outcome. Finally a history of leg pain of six months or less is associated with a higher success rate compared to those with a longer history.

4. The 'problem' of back pain and spasm

This has been reported in up to 40% of patients following chemonucleolysis and is self-limiting. Back pain has been studied in several prospective randomised studies. Comparing chemonucleolysis and surgery in general shows little if any difference in the incidence. Randomised studies comparing low dose chemonucleolysis to standard dose in which back pain was looked at very carefully have been carried out to see if low dose was as effective as standard dose and compared the incidence of back pain[42,43].

A Single-blind Parallel-group Study was performed to compare the Efficacy of Low Dose versus Standard Dose Intradiscal Chymopapain (DISCASE) in the treatment of herniated intervertebral disc disease[43]. Twelve patients received the low dose (2 ml containing 2.5 nkat chymopapain) and ten patients received the standard dose (2 ml containing 5.0 nkat chymopapain). Three patients reported a total of four adverse events (back pain and/or leg pain), one of the patients being on low dose treatment. There were no withdrawals from the study. Low dose patients had lower pain levels, particularly for back pain in the two days following chemonucleolysis, but the difference was not statistically significant. Low dose patients also required less analgesia post-operatively. At day 14 after the operation there was a significant difference in favour of low dose patients in the change from baseline in the Roland-Morris functional assessment score. By day 42 there was no difference between the treatment groups in either the investigator's or patients' assessments of treatment effectiveness. Overall, chemonucleolysis was judged to be successful in 83% of the low dose patients and in 80% of the standard patients. This study strongly suggests that low dose chemonucleolysis is as effective as standard dose with lower levels of post-operative pain and significantly less disability at 14 days. Only two patients (10%) had significant back pain attributable to the procedure.

Salam in 1991, suggested that injection of Marcaine following chemonucleolysis would reduce the incidence of back pain and/or muscle spasm. A prospective, randomised, double blind study was set up to evaluate this hypothesis[44].

Thirty-six patients were randomly allocated into three groups each of 12 patients. Group 1 had no injection carried out following chemonucleolysis. Group 2 had a para-discal injection of 10 ml of normal saline. Group 3 had an injection of 10 ml 0.25% Marcaine. Chemonucleolysis was carried out using the 2 needle technique. The large outer needle was inserted down to the edge of the annulus of the injected disc. On removal of the central needle the outer needle was left in position and the Marcaine/saline injection given through this needle. Seven millilitres of injection were given para-discally and the other 3 ml injected as the needle was withdrawn. Back pain and leg pain were assessed on a 9-point scale on days 1,2,3,4,5,6,7,14,28 and 42 following injection. Standardized analgesic intake was monitored. Disability was assessed using the Roland Morris questionnaire at day 1 pre-injection and days 14, 28 and 42 post injection. The final result was deemed either a success or failure by the Surgeon and patient separately using the 6-point rating scale. All the data were entered into a computer database for analysis. Preliminary examination of this data already indicated that the severity of post-injection pain may be dependant, at least in part, upon back pain experienced prior to the chemonucleolysis procedure. Full analysis of the results is not yet available but it appears evident that Marcaine reduces the post-injection pain or discomfort during the 8 hours post procedure. It is anticipated that the findings will extend the present knowledge of the basis of post-chemonucleolysis back pain.

5. Relative indications (or contraindications)

Not all patients have clear indications for *any* form of treatment and chemonucleolysis is no exception.

1. Previous chemonucleolysis. Repeat injections to the same or another disc have yielded results comparable to repeat surgery. Premedication with H_1 and H_2 blockers or pre-treatment testing to exclude sensitised patients is recommended.

2. Spondylolisthesis. Excellent and good results have been obtained in treating disc herniations causing sciatica in this group.

3. Sequestration. It is clear from my own study that half sequestrated discs do respond.

4. Epidural leakage. During discography one frequently sees the dye pass into a protrusion, occasionally behind the posterior longitudinal ligament or even into the epidural space. There is no evidence that Chymopapain in any of these situations causes damage. Conventional wisdom is that if there is a risk of dye escaping into the epidural space then chemonucleolysis should not be carried out. The main value of discography is that it will demonstrate, by immediate escape of contrast into the cerebrospinal fluid where it rapidly disperses, the tiny proportion of patients who have an intradural protrusion and therefore are at risk from intradural leakage of Chymopapain. This is an absolute contra-indication to injection of Chymopapain.

5. Long duration of history. Patients with a history of leg pain of more than six months have been shown to have a significantly reduced response rate. However some patients when counselled take the view that if they can avoid surgery by accepting a procedure that is ten times safer than surgery overall, and even at a potential success rate something under 60%, that the procedure is worthwhile.

6. Spinal stenosis. Porter *et al.*[45] demonstrated that in young mining recruits and nurses that there is a normal variation in the oblique diameter of the spinal canal. His findings, carried out by the use of ultrasound, were confirmed anatomically[46]. The ultrasound readings of a group of patients who had come to disc enucleation for sciatica demonstrated that they all were within the tenth percentile of the smallest oblique diameter[47]. Clearly the diagnosis of spinal stenosis is in the perception of the surgeon or radiologist reporting. If a patient has the classical symptoms and signs of sciatica, that is dominant leg pain and reduced straight leg raising with or without paraesthesia and neurological findings and with a positive investigation indicating clearly a disc protrusion compatible with the patient's symptoms and signs then this is an indication for chemonucleolysis.

7. Workman's compensation. Many studies have clearly shown, particularly from the USA, that such patients have a significantly lower success rate than patients who are self-employed or in employment.

8. Calcification in the protrusion. It is the author's experience that a protrusion with speckled calcification or calcification within an acute disc herniation is

likely to be similar to acute calcification in other situations where the
material is soft, like 'toothpaste'. A large proportion of these protrusions do
respond to chemonucleolysis in the same way as any other soft disc
herniation. However, clear cut long term calcification secondary to
osteophyte formation is less likely to respond to chemonucleolysis.

6. Absolute contraindications

1.   Rapidly progressive neurological deficit. Clearly immediate surgical
         decompression is the treatment of choice. However, on two occasions a
         situation has arisen where the surgical theatre was not likely to be available
         for several hours and a chemonucleolysis was performed in these
         circumstances in the X-ray Department under sedation and local anaesthesia,
         with relief of patient's symptoms and neurological recovery (Personal
         Communication).
2.   Bladder and bowel dysfunction. It is the author's opinion that even the
         smallest evidence of bladder and bowel dysfunction in the presence of a very
         large protrusion, requires surgical decompression. In the one case of cauda
         equina syndrome in retrospect the patient admitted on direct questioning to
         have minor bladder dysfunction in the form of hesitancy and reduced control.
         Clearly with such large protrusions, a relatively small increase in size of the
         protrusion caused by increased intradiscal pressure following injection of
         chemonucleolysis may be the cause.
3.   History of allergy. A known history of allergy to Chymopapain and papaya
         is potentially an absolute contra-indication because of the increased risk of
         anaphylaxis. Pre-medication with steroid and H_1 and H_2 blockers are advised
         but are probably unlikely to prevent an anaphylactic reaction because of the
         nature of the process. At best they may reduce its severity. A history of
         atopy has been shown to have no correlation with allergy to
         chemonucleolysis.
4.   Positive sensitivity test. Skin testing, Chymofast and RAST tests for
         Chymopapain if positive are excluded from published series. They are small
         in numbers in the general population in Europe and those remaining patients
         have a very low anaphylaxis or reaction rate following Chymopapain
         injection. The author's experience of the RAST test (in preparation) in over
         200 cases has not shown any clear cut correlation between positivity on
         RAST testing and reaction. One case of anaphylaxis out of 1,300 patients
         occurred in a patient who was RAST negative.

7. Other important indications

1.   The adolescent disc. This is relatively rare compared to adult disc herniation
         and results are comparable to the results of surgery

2. Patients greater than 60. Both the population and different anatomical sites age at different rates. Clearly, acute disc herniations do occur in older people and do respond to treatment at least as well as in other age groups[40,41].

3. Recurrence after surgery. Some of Lyman Smith's first published series of chemonucleolyses were performed on patients previously treated by surgery. He and others have obtained good results comparable to surgery. Surgery is more difficult due to scarring present from previous surgery and therefore complications are likely to be greater. Chemonucleolysis is the same straightforward procedure.

4. Lateral herniations. The small published series suggest a success rate of 80%.

5. Cervical disc herniation. Chymopapain chemonucleolysis for acute cervical soft disc herniation has now been shown to have dramatically good results[49].

8. Anaphylaxis

The incidence is 0.5-0.1% in the USA and 0.02% in Europe. Anaphylaxis is a perfectly treatable condition. All doctors and surgeons engaged in any hospital procedures should know how to treat it. The procedure should only be done when the appropriate equipment and medication is immediately available to the operator. In this situation anaphylaxis if it occurs is treatable and the patient should survive. The occurrence of anaphylaxis has no effect on the result of chemonucleolysis[50].

9. Neurological complications

Adverse events such as transverse myelitis, cauda equina syndrome, meningeal haemorrhage and epilepsy have been described as complications[50]. However, the excellent review carried out by Nordby, Wright and Schofield[51] showed that the adverse event reported to the FDA during the first 10 years of reintroduction of chemonucleolysis into the United States was of an incidence of 0.09%, that is 121 cases in 135,000 patients. There were 7 cases of fatal anaphylaxis, 24 cases of infection, 32 cases of haemorrhage, 32 cases of neurological sequelae and 15 miscellaneous reported events. They compared their results including anaphylaxis with surgical complications encountered in 23,395 cases treated by 'laminectomy' in community hospital patients[52]. The overall complication rate in the surgery cases was double that of the Chymopapain treated patients. The mortality in the surgical group was three times the chemonucleolysis group and if one excludes anaphylaxis, then the overall complication rate is 12 times greater in the surgical group. Bouillet[53] reported surgical complications occurring in specialist centres throughout Europe in patients treated by surgery and chemonucleolysis. The overall complication rate in the surgical group was 10 times that of the chemonucleolysis group as was the serious complication rate, and the complications requiring treatment were approximately six times greater in the surgery group. My own complications, recorded in a series of 1,300 cases, show an overall complication rate of 0.36%.

10. Relationship of result to protrusion size

Postacchini suggests that severe symptoms along with large herniations do not do better than surgery but there is no consensus on this. In general symptoms resolve as the hernia shrinks and *vice versa* but this is not consistent.

11. Cost-effectiveness

Many authors have in the USA shown significantly reduced costs comparing chemonucleolysis to surgery taking all factors into account including further surgery[54,55]. The cost of primary disc enucleation of a lumbar intervertebral disc in an NHS hospital in Aberdeen is now £2,121 compared with that of chemonucleolysis of £998. This means that even if all disc herniations were treated primarily by chemonucleolysis with 20% requiring further surgery, the overall costs would still be 25% less. Within the National Health Service surgeons and units are valued according to the throughput of patients. A simple calculation of the time required to carry out 1,300 chemonucleolysis procedures over 11 years shows that substituting surgery in the form of disc enucleation would require another year and three months, and allowing for other surgical procedures, I would require another six years and three months just to complete these 1,300 cases.

Percutaneous discectomy has been popular in recent years. However, recent results published suggest that it is significantly less successful than chemonucleolysis in treating disc herniation. Also, the potential complications such as major vascular injury, infection, cauda equina and root damage are significantly greater[56].

12. Conclusions

I must conclude therefore that chemonucleolysis is a procedure that has withstood the test of time. As far as the patient and the surgeon is concerned it is simple and safe compared to other methods of treatment. It is equally efficacious as surgery, the gold-standard treatment, if the patients are selected correctly. In this modern world of economics and cost cutting it is certainly economical. Finally, there is no doubt that relief of symptoms means a lasting long term result.

13. References

1.   D. Wardlaw, The Case For Chemonucleolysis. *Orthopaedics*. In Press
2.   E.F. Jansen and A.K. Balls, *J. Biol. Chem.* **137** (1941) 459.
3.   L. Smith, P.J. Garvin, R.M. Gesler and R.B. Jennings, *Nature* **198** (1963) 1311.
4.   L. Smith, *J.A.M.A.* **187** (1964) 137.
5.   I. Macnab, J.A. McCulloch, D.S. Weiner, E.P. Hugo, R.D. Galway and D. Dall, *Canad. J. Surg.* **14** (1971) 280.
6.   E.J. Nordby and G.L. Lucas, *Clin. Orthop.* **90** (1973) 119.

7. J.A. McCulloch, *J. Bone Joint Surg.* **59-A** (1977) 45.
8. B.M. Onofrio, *J. Neurosurg.* **42** (1975) 384.
9. C. Watts, G. Hutchinson, J. Stern and K. Clark, *J. Neurosurg.* **42** (1975) 397.
10. E.J. Dabezies and M. Brunet, *Orthopedics.* **1** (1978) 26.
11. P.R. Schwetschenau, A. Ramirez, J. Johnston, C. Wiggs and A.N. Martins, *J. Neurosurg.* **45** (1976) 622.
12. A.N. Martins, A. Ramirez, J. Johnston, P.R. Schwetschenau, *J. Neurosurg.* **49** (1978) 816.
13. R.D. Fraser, *Spine* **7** (1982) 608.
14. R.D. Fraser, *Spine* **9** (1984) 815.
15. M.J. Javid, E.J. Nordby, L.T. Ford, *et al.*, *J.A.M.A.* **249** (1983) 2489.
16. E.J. Dabezies, K. Langford, J. Morris, C.B. Sheilds and H.A. Wilkinson, *Spine* **13** (1988) 561.
17. J. Feldman, C.J. Menkes, G. Pallardy *et al.*, *Rev. Rhum. Mal. Osteoartic.* **53** (1986) 147.
18. D.J. McDermott, K. Agre, M. Brim, *et al.*, *Spine* **10** (1985) 242.
19. M.J. Javid, *J. Neurosurg.* **62** (1985) 662.
20. D. Parkinson, *J. Neurosurg.* **59** (1983) 990.
21. N. Flanagan and L. Smith, *Clin. Orthop.* **206** (1986) 15.
22. E.J. Nordby, *Clin. Orthop.* **206** (1986) 2.
23. R.J. Maciunas, B.M. Onofrio, *Clin. Orthop.* **206** (1986) 37.
24. F. Mansfield, K. Polivy, R. Boyd and J. Huddleston, *Clin. Orthop.* **206** (1986) 67.
25. J. Weinstein, K.F. Spratt, T. Lehmann, T. McNeill and W. Hejna, *J. Bone Joint Surg.* **68-A** (1986) 43.
26. W.J. Gogan, R.D. Fraser, *Spine* **17** (1992) 388.
27. H. Weber, *Spine* **8** (1983) 131.
28. D. Wardlaw, I.K. Ritchie and C. Eastmond, Chemonucleolysis compared to surgery: A prospective randomised study in 100 patients. Read at the *Second Annual Meeting of the International Intradiscal Therapy Society*, Orlando, Florida, 1989.
29. J.A. McCulloch and I. Macnab, *Sciatica and chymopapain.* (Williams & Wilkins, Baltimore, 1983).
30. J.A. McCulloch and G. Waddell, *Br. J. Radiol.* **51** (1978) 498.
31. I.J. Stern, *Clin. Orthop.* **67** (1969) 42.
32. A.A. Kapsalis, I.J. Stern and I. Bornstein, *J. Lab. Clin. Med.* **83** (1974) 532.
33. P. Dolan, M.A. Adams, W.C. Hutton, *J. Bone Joint Surg.* **69-B** (1987) 422.
34. D. Wardlaw, I.K. Ritchie and C. Eastmond, Radiological analysis of Prospective randomised study of chemonucleolysis compared to surgery in 100 patients. Read at the *Third Annual Meeting of the International Intradiscal Therapy Society*, p70, Marbella, Spain, 1990.
35. F. Postacchini, R. Lami and M. Massobrio, *Spine* **12** (1987) 87.
36. R. Bouillet, *Acta Orthop. Belg.* **49** (1983) 48.

37. C. Crawshaw, A.M. Frazer, W.F. Merriam, R.C. Mulholland and J.K. Webb, *Spine* **9** (1984) 87.
38. A.H. Alexander, J.K. Burkus, J.B. Mitchell, W.V. Ayers, *Clin. Orthop.* **244** (1989) 158.
39. A. Deburge, J. Rocolle and M. Benoist, *Spine* **10** (1985) 812.
40. M. Benoist, H. Parent, B. Lassale, A. Deburge, Lumbar disc herniation in the elderly. A study of long term results of chemonucleolysis. Read at the *Fifth Annual Meeting of the International Intradiscal Therapy Society*, Nice, France, 1992.
41. R. Deutman, H. Douma, Chemonucleolysis in the patient aged 60 years or more. Read at the Read at the *First Annual Meeting of the International Intradiscal Therapy Society*, Fort Lauderdale, Florida, 1988.
42. J.F.A. Bonneville, A randomised double blind study comparing lowdose (2000 units) to standard dose (4000 units) Chymodiactin in the treatment of herniated lumbar intervertebral discs. Read at the *Fourth Annual Meeting of the International Intradiscal Therapy Society*, Houston, Texas, 1991.
43. D. Wardlaw, A single blind parallel group study to compare lowdose and standard dose Chymopapain in herniated intervertebral disc disease. Read at the *Fourth Annual Meeting of the International Intradiscal Therapy Society*, Houston, Texas 1991.
44. R Murali, D. Wardlaw, P. Nie, *The role of 0.25% Bipivocaine in the relief of post-chemonucleolysis back pain. *(A double-blind parallel group study to compare the efficacy and reliability of). Read at the *Seventh Annual Meeting of the International Intradiscal Therapy Society*, Aberdeen, Scotland, UK, 1994.
45. R.W. Porter, M. Wicks and D. Ottewell, *J. Bone Joint Surg.* **60-B** (1978) 481.
46. R. Kadziolka, M. Asztély, K. Hanai, T. Hansson and A. Nachemson, *J. Bone Joint Surg.* **63-B** (1981) 504.
47. R.W. Porter, M. Wicks and D. Ottewell, *J. Bone Joint Surg.* **60-B** (1978) 485.
48. J. Richaud, Y. Lazorthes, J.C. Verdie, A. Bonafe, *Acta Neurochir.* **91** (1988) 116.
49. F. Gomez-Cassestrana, Cervical chemonucleolysis. Three years of experience. Read at the *Fourth Annual Meeting of the International Intradiscal Therapy Society*, Houston, Texas, USA, 1991.
50. K. Agre, R.R. Wilson, M. Brim and D.J. McDermott, *Spine* **9** (1984) 479.
51. E.J. Nordby, P.H. Wright and S.R. Schofield, *Clin. Orthop.* **293** (1993) 122.
52. L.F. Ramirez and R. Thisted, *Neurosurgery.* **25** (1989) 226.
53. R. Bouillet, *Clin. Orthop.* **251** (1990) 144.
54. L.F. Ramirez and M.J. Javid, *Spine* **10** (1985) 363.
55. R. Sancho Navarro, C. Ardila Guervo and R. Ramos Escalona, *Review of Orthopaedic Trauma.* **34** (1990) 588.
56. M. Revel, C. Payan, C. Vallee *et al.*, *Spine* **18** (1993) 1.

CHAPTER 19

LUMBOSACRAL AND SPONDYLO-PELVIC ARTHRODESIS

AN ALTERNATIVE CONCEPT IN THE SURGICAL MANAGEMENT OF LUMBAR DEGENERATIVE DISC DISEASE: FLEXIBLE STABILISATION

A.D.H. Gardner

1. Introduction

This chapter explores the concept that flexible stabilisation of a spinal motion segment is not only effective in relieving intractable pain and disability in degenerative disc disease but is also a quicker, less invasive and more physiological method than conventional bone grafting with or without instrumentation (Figure 1).

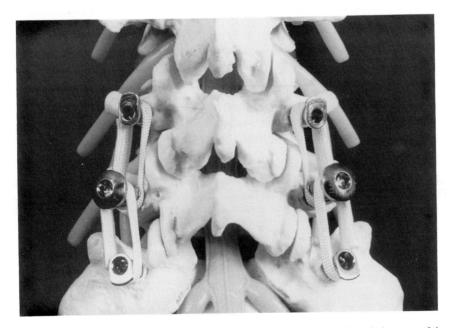

Figure 1. The plastic model shows the Graf implant in place. Note the relatively lateral placement of the pedicle screws to keep the bands clear of the facet joints. If there is impingement on the facet joint the prominent bone should be osteotomised to prevent chafing. This technique depends on posterior element and facet joint integrity to achieve stabilisation. It is therefore less suitable for isthmic spondylolisthesis, especially greater than grade 1.

Bone grafting to achieve complete abolition of movement and secure fixation of the lumbosacral junction should, if carried out successfully on appropriate patients, produce near 100% good or excellent results in patients with intolerable low back pain from degenerative disc disease. The operative word here is 'should' because all of us, without exception, who have significant experience in this difficult field of surgery are aware that there is a distressingly high failure rate with dissatisfied patients running at 20% to 40% of the total depending on the author[2,3,7,8,17,21,22,25,27,29,30].

Although the above figures are not entirely satisfactory, they do indicate that a large number of individuals can be returned to a tolerable and useful life at the peak of their economic activity (the mean age in most series is around 40 years). These patients have usually tried every other modality of treatment and would otherwise have to settle for a life of significant disability, although some may improve with time while others worsen.

It is important at this stage to distinguish between the results of spinal fusion in degenerative disc disease and the results in spondylolisthesis. Some patients do, of course, have both.

Some papers reporting the results of spinal arthrodesis contain a mixture of patients suffering from degenerative disc disease and spondylolisthesis, mixing the good results of the latter with the less satisfactory results of the former. This confusion should be avoided in outcome studies of these two very different conditions[31].

Patients suffering from L5 spondylolisthesis, whether isthmic or otherwise, have a much better prognosis following surgery with around 80% to 90% satisfaction. A demonstrable failure of fusion on lateral flexion and extension x-rays is sometimes compatible with a good result. This is in marked contrast to patients suffering from degenerative disc disease in whom failure of fusion usually means that they are the same or worse than before surgery, having the pain from their pseudoarthrosis in addition to their original pain source.

Such contrasting outcomes between the two conditions leads to the logical conclusion that the pain sources in spondylolisthesis and degenerative disc disease are in many ways different. They just happen to share the same surgical remedy namely spinal arthrodesis.

Our knowledge of the origin of pain in mechanical disorders of the lumbosacral junction is still undeveloped. The main evidence comes from anatomical and histological studies of the sites of concentration of unmyelinated nerve fibres[1,36], from injection studies[15], from spinal probing[28] and from discography[32]. These sites include the subchondral area of the vertebral end plates, the outer layers of the annulus fibrosus, the anterior and posterior longitudinal ligaments[18], the facet joint capsules[6] and the soft tissues surrounding the motion segment[4,14].

In spondylolisthesis it is quite possible that the isthmic defect and also the abnormally loaded and hypermobile L5/S1 facet joints may be major pain sources[35]. Abolition of this hypermobility by fusion or a strong fibrous pseudoarthrosis may be sufficient to abolish symptoms, whereas in degenerative disc disease the main pain source may be largely from the disc itself which requires an alteration of loading as much as immobilisation before symptoms are abolished. A failed fusion certainly does not achieve the former although it may achieve the latter to some extent.

To summarise, the pain sources in isthmic spondylolisthesis may well be mainly in the posterior column, whereas in degenerative disc disease we know from discographic studies that the anterior column is frequently a major pain source. There are, of course, overlaps with discogenic pain in some spondylolistheses, and facet joint pain in association with symptomatic degenerate discs.

Being dissatisfied with the results of spinal fusion for low back pain, Professor Pierre Senegas of Bordeaux and then Henry Graf of Lyon set about the development of a flexible stabilisation system using polypropylene tape to produce stabilisation of painful degenerate discs.

Initially Senegas tried taping the spinous processes of the lower lumbar vertebrae together with and without spacers to produce stability but he has never been sufficiently satisfied with the outcome of this procedure to advocate its general use.

In the mid 1980s Henry Graf of Lyon, France, started work on an implant system using titanium pedicle screws with polyester bands of varying sizes in order to produce strong bilateral stabilisation of the motion segment. Eventually, preliminary results of clinical implantation of the pedicle screw and band system were sufficiently encouraging to persuade Dr. Graf to carry out flexible stabilisation as the procedure of choice in patients with severe lumbar backache[10]. He obtained his best results in patients with degenerative disc disease. Those with spondylolisthesis were also satisfactory but those with significant scoliosis had poor results[11]. Initially, there were some technical problems with band breakage due to chafing on the facet joints, and screw breakage[12]. The former was solved by osteotomising any impingeing part of the facet joint and the latter by strengthening the shaft-thread junction of the pedicle screw in 1991, since when there have been virtually no screw breakages after many thousands of implantations[12].

2. Philosophy and mode of action

The precise mode of action of the Graf flexible stabilisation system is not yet fully understood. However, its efficacy in patients with intolerable pain from degenerative disc disease is, in my view and in the view of an increasing number of colleagues, sufficiently well established to encourage its use in well selected patients in whom the outcome is prospectively and systematically recorded.

The possible modes of action are:

> i) Immobilisation in extension providing stability through coaptation of the facet joints (Figure 2).
> ii) Alteration of annular and endplate load bearing.
> iii) Posterior annular compression resulting in
> > a) closure of annular tears
> > b) elimination of neo-innervation and neo-vascularisation
> iv) Splinting of the motion segment to allow healing of damaged tissues
> v) Band relaxation over the first four to six months allowing some return of movement.

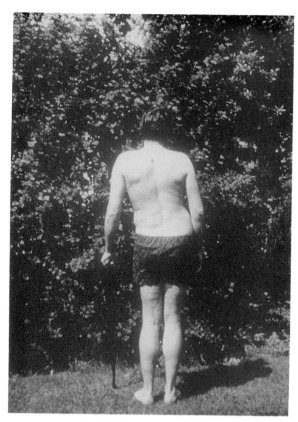

Figure 2. 40 year old man with 'sciatic' scoliosis. This man had intermittent attacks of severe lumbar spasm but no leg pain. Lumbar muscle spasm results in immobilisation in extension but he did not require surgery for his lumbar instability syndrome. Muscle spasm results in immobilisation of the painful motion segments in extension which is the natural position of spinal stability.

The question is commonly asked, and it is most important to appreciate, that the combined effect of immobilisation of a motion segment in extension may result in significant narrowing of the foraminal outlet of that segmental nerve, both by infolding of ligamentum flavum and facet joint capsule and also by approximation of the superior articular process and the pedicle forming the boundaries of the bony canal at that level. (Figure 3) Also there may be a small additional degree of retrolisthesis of the upper vertebral body on the lower which could cause some lateral recess compression to the nerve root of the lower level.

It is, therefore, essential that if there is any suspicion of foraminal or lateral recess stenosis, not only on the symptomatic side but also on the asymptomatic side, then a flavectomy or undercutting facetectomy must be carried out.

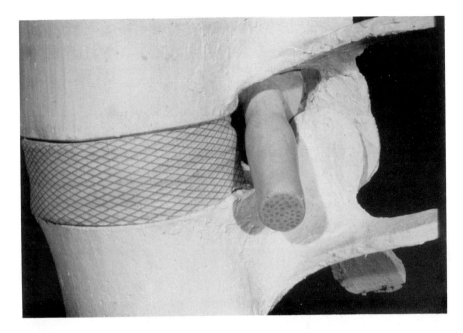

Figure 3. This model indicates the borders of the neural foramen. In full extension the superior articular process may impinge on the foramen, especially if there is disc narrowing or bone or soft tissue hypertrophy.

One of the commonest complications in my first 50 cases was radicular pain in 12 patients[12]. This subsided spontaneously over a few weeks in all but 4 who needed further decompressive surgery. These patients were all much relieved of their back pain but their radicular symptoms of sensory disturbance and paraesthesia were certainly a nuisance. Two patients had motor disturbance, one with some dorsiflexion weakness, the other had weak quadriceps. I will now discuss each of these mechanisms in more detail.

2.1. Immobilisation in extension giving facet joint stability

The application of the appropriate sized polyester (Dacrilene) bands to the bilateral pedicle screws under moderate tension, (20-40 N on the scale of the special measuring instrument in females and 40-60 N in males), immobilises the motion segment in extension. This has the effect of locking the facet joints and abolishing the rotatory and flexion-extension hypermobility readily observed at surgery.

Immobilisation in extension also restores the lumbar lordosis which has been lost through shortening of the anterior column (Figure 4).

A strain gauged calliper is under development to provide objective measurement of these movements. After band application the motion segment is virtually immobile with a surprising degree of stability.

2.2. *Alteration of annular and endplate load bearing*

It is well established that there are unmyelinated nerve endings in the outer layers of the annulus fibrosis, the sub-chondral bone adjacent to the end plates and in the anterior and posterior longitudinal ligaments. All these nerve endings are presumably involved in what is commonly known as discogenic pain. In addition, the facet joint capsules and the surrounding soft tissues also contain pain sensitive nerve endings and presumably contribute to the overall pain syndrome. Some experienced clinicians believe that facet joint pain is of dominating importance but others favour discogenic pain. No doubt the lumbar instability syndrome is a combination of the two but I believe that discogenic pain, as detected by discography, predominates. In a minority of cases, provocative discography is not helpful, perhaps because facet joint pain is not demonstrated by this technique.

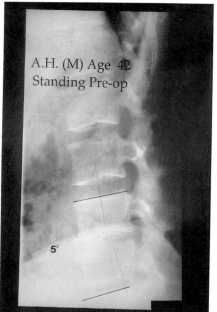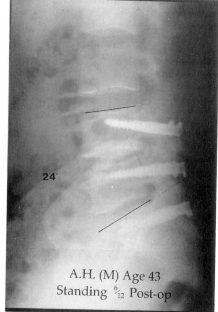

Figure 4 (a)-(b).This man had a stooping posture prior to surgery which was fully corrected post-operatively long term. He remains very greatly improved 3 years from the time of surgery.

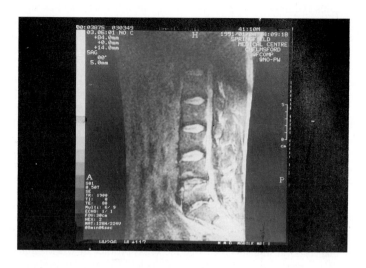

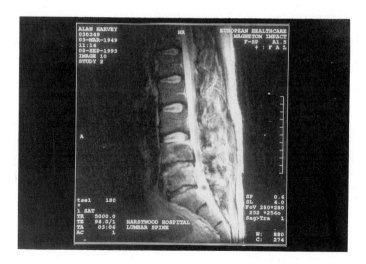

Figure 4 (c)-(d). The same patient agreed to a further MRI scan for research purposes 2 years 8 months after his pre-operative MRI. There has been no significant alteration in the Modic changes on either side of the L.4/5 disc.

Spinal fusion, by achieving rigid immobilisation, will relieve loading on the facet joints, the annulus and the end plates in the majority of cases but, undoubtedly, there are some patients in whom the small amount of movement still present after posterior or intertransverse fusion, continues to produce symptoms, perhaps through continuing loading of the sensitive end plates[24]. In these patients anterior fusion is sometimes successful[33].

Loading of the disc has been investigated by the technique of stress profilometry[20]. This technique measures the distribution of compressive stress throughout the annulus and nucleus of a cadaveric disc. A miniature pressure transducer mounted on a needle is inserted into a disc and pressure readings are taken on withdrawal. A stress profile is produced corresponding to the 'functional' annulus and nucleus.

An L4/5 cadaver motion segment was mounted in dental plaster and secured in a computer controlled servo-hydraulic materials testing machine. The specimen was loaded to 500 newtons and 2000 newtons (which correspond to the compressive forces during standing and light manual labour) in pure compression and flexion. Stress profiles were measured. The Graf stabilisation system was applied to the specimen and the process was repeated.

The experiment was repeated on another motion segment and the results were similar. It was found that the Graf implants increased the stress profiles by 0.3 MPa in both load situations. This represents approximately a 50% increase in annular loading after Graf instrumentation. It is suggested, therefore, that restoration of annular loading may be an important effect of Graf stabilisation.

2.3. Closure of annular tears

Where there is an established annular leak into the epidural space demonstrated on discography, this can be confirmed by saline injection at the time of surgery. If the intra-discal needle is left in place until after the Graf bands have been applied and further injection is then attempted, it will be found that the annular tear no longer leaks. This has been confirmed in all five patients in whom it has been tried. On the other hand, a cruciate incision made in the annulus for removing the disc contents continues to leak after the application of the bands. Perhaps because it gives a much more direct access to the interior of the disc in both longitudinal and horizontal planes whereas an annular leak is assumed to have a more serpentine course through the annulus. This finding suggests that application of the Graf bands results in closure of annular leaks and less complete tears by compression of the posterior annulus.

2.4. Posterior annular compression

Possibly as a result of a fall in intra-discal pressure, neo-vascularisation and neo-innervation are thought to occur in some abnormally painful discs, particularly involving the unloaded and possibly torn posterior annulus. Re-loading of the annulus will compress the abnormal nerve endings and capillaries out of existence. Closure of the annular tear as described above will prevent the passage of irritant breakdown products from the disc space into the well innervated outer layers of the annulus and the epidural space.

It seems that the combined effect of these mechanisms, and perhaps others, may restore a painful abnormally mobile (perhaps 10% are hypermobile) and degenerate disc to the much more common state of a stable, relatively painless degenerate disc which is so commonly observed on x-rays of the adult lumbar spine and is of little clinical significance. To use video terminology, it is possible that Graf stabilisation 'fast-forwards' the natural history of a painful 'unstable disc' to that of a relatively painless 'stable disc' so commonly found from middle age onwards according to the philosophy of Kirkaldy-Willis[16].

2.5. Early motion segment splinting

Once the Graf instrumentation is in place, the motion segment is virtually immobile in full extension. However, *in-vitro* testing indicates that the band will stretch by about 15% within the first week. This will even out any differences of tension on the two sides and allow the spine and the implant to 'bed down' together with a little movement.

This splinting effect results in rapid stiffening of the motion segment in the same way as an injured knee stiffens after immobilisation in plaster of Paris. This has been confirmed in several patients who have had to be re-explored after 4-6 weeks to relieve foraminal compression. After detachment of the bands from the screws it is quite difficult to open up the inter-laminar space, even using a vertebral spreader, in order to carry out an undercutting facetectomy. This occurs at levels noted to be markedly hypermobile at initial surgery.

2.6. Late band relaxation and partial movement return

In-vitro testing further indicates that the bands will stretch by 10% - 15% more between the first week and 4 - 6 months. During this time there is usually a millimetre or two of measurable disc narrowing due to posterior annular compression. This will further de-tension the bands so that there is no longer any strain on the pedicle screws or bands and therefore no tendency to late breakage. The bands remain *in situ* as loose 'check ligaments' to guard against any excessive and damaging movement. This has been observed on occasional re-operation for late blood-born infection a year or two post-operatively when the implant has had to be removed. All six patients have retained their good results so far up to three years after implant removal.

Although the inelastic radio opaque marker threads often break after a few months, I have experienced only one definite band breakage in over 300 cases, this was probably due to chafing against the facet joint. No screw breakage has occurred since the screw-thread junction was strengthened in 1991.

3. Indication for Graf stabilisation

Given the present state of knowledge, the prime indication for Graf stabilisation is degenerative disc disease with lumbar instability syndrome. Degenerative disc disease may be evident on plain x-ray but younger patients will often be equally symptomatic with normal plain x-rays.

MRI scanning showing disc dehydration is the investigation of choice but needs careful interpretation. A small number of patients, often those in their twenties, have a normal MRI scan but provocative discography indicates discogenic pain.

Lumbar instability syndrome may be defined as a state of mainly midline chronic low back pain with acute exacerbations and/or muscle spasm on certain movements, not caused by radicular pain although this may additionally be present in some patients.

It will be observed that as the duration of low back pain increases from months to years, the pain referral pattern becomes wider, sometimes spreading up between the shoulder blades to the occiput and down one or both legs in a non-dermatomal distribution, sometimes as far as the foot, usually to the metatarsal area of the sole. At the same time, spinal buttock and thigh muscles and ligaments show increasing pain and tenderness and their attachments to bone also become symptomatic. These latter secondary effects often take many months to settle and sometimes they may cause long term symptoms after Graf stabilisation has abolished the acute instability symptoms and the midline back pain.

4. The lumbar instability syndrome

The term 'lumbar instability syndrome', being a clinical entity, does not require the demonstration of a measurable radiological shift which is usually disappointingly absent on lateral flexion and extension x-rays. The syndrome has little to do with the radiological entity of 'lumbar instability' as defined by White & Panjabi[34].

Henry Graf has described the CT twist test in which gapping of the facet joints of the affected level can be demonstrated in some patients on CT scanning with the patient in a position of spinal rotation. It is not known what percentage of asymptomatic patients would demonstrate facet joint gapping or what percentage of symptomatic patients have too much pain and spasm preventing sufficient rotation to produce gapping.

Four types of lumbar instability syndrome can be recognised:

Type A)   Degenerative overt. The clinical syndrome, as described above, is present, along with obvious disc disease on plain x-ray. These patients are predominantly middle aged with an equal sex ratio.

Type B)   Degenerative covert. The lumbar instability syndrome is present but with normal plain x-ray. MRI and/or discography is required to demonstrate the pain source. These are predominantly female patients in their twenties and thirties and represent about 25% of those in the operated series[9].

Type C)   Post-prolapse instability. There has been a previous history of severe radicular pain. This may have been treated:
        i) with surgery
        ii) without surgery
The back pain by itself is disabling apart from the sciatica (Figure 5).

Type D)   Stiff segment instability
        i) adjacent to a previous spinal fusion (Figure 6)
        ii) adjacent to a congenital stiff segment such as a transitional L5 vertebra.

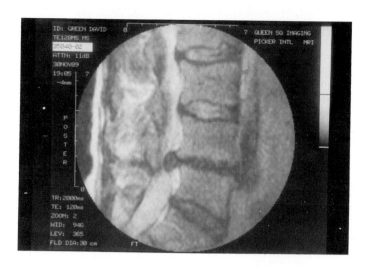

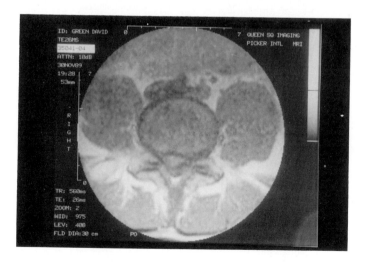

Figure 5. This 50 year old man had a 15 year history of increasingly disabling low back pain with the onset of severe radicular pain with neurological signs six weeks previously. Discectomy alone, while relieving his sciatica, would in all probability have left him with unacceptable back pain.

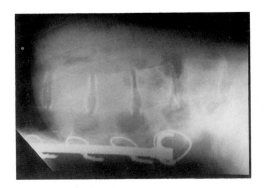

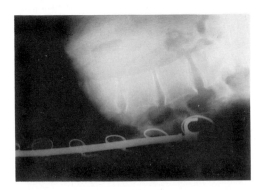

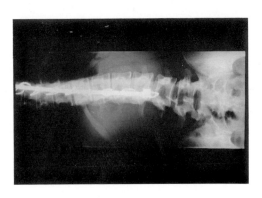

Figure 6. Radiographs of a 23 year old female who had undergone successful Harrington-Luque surgery nine years previously. For two years she had experienced increasing mid-lumbar backache with no obvious cause. (b) is taken in flexion and (c) in extension. The L3/4 disc is clearly hypermobile. There is some fixed kyphosis at L2/3.

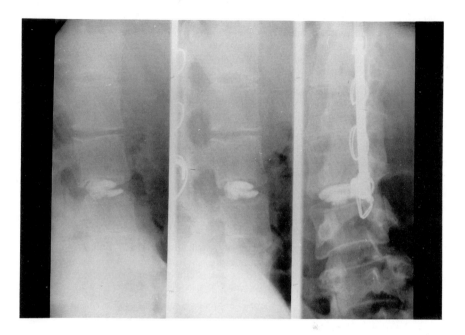

Figure 6(d). The discogram is morphologically normal but her pain was reproduced. This is a good indication for Graf flexible stabilisation rather than a further fusion.

In summary, the ideal patient for Graf stabilisation is one in whom there is a characteristic history of lumbar instability syndrome not responding to the usual non-operative measures and in whom there is sufficient disability with loss of quality of life to justify surgery. The patient is not unduly distressed, has not been severely disabled for more than a year and is not seeking compensation.

The outcome does not seem to be significantly affected by the degree of disability, a single episode of previous disc surgery, the absence or presence of obvious disc degeneration unless extreme, the age or sex of the patient so long as they are reasonably physically fit, or the number of levels instrumented.

Factors contra-indicating a Graf stabilisation are a symptomatic pseudoarthrosis from a previous fusion, obvious osteoporosis, isthmic spondylolisthesis (although Grade 1 may be acceptable), or degenerative spondylolisthesis in excess of Grade 1.

5. Investigations

It goes without saying that all patients must have had a thorough course of all the conservative modalities of treatment likely to be effective prior to the consideration of surgery. It is also emerging that, in common with other series of surgically treated patients with degenerative disc disease, those with prolonged disability prior to surgery, patients showing undue distress and patients involved in compensation do less well after Graf stabilisation. The severity of disability does not seem to be prognostically significant provided it is of relatively recent onset, *i.e.* less than one year of severe disability.

All candidates for Graf surgery should have a thorough clinical evaluation. The clinical history provides 80% of the data and will indicate whether or not the patient is a candidate for surgery. Invariably the back pain is worse than the leg pain unless there has been a recent acute disc prolapse with a previous history of increasingly intolerable back pain. The back pain : leg pain ratio (*e.g.* 70 : 30) is an important item to record.

All patients should record a visual analogue pain scale and a pain drawing. The Oswestry Disability Index is widely used, along with a measure of psychological factors such as the MSPQ Zung scale and the SF36 measurement of health perception[23].

All patients should undergo MRI investigation as this is the standard investigation of choice prior to Graf stabilisation. The MRI scan does not, of course, show pain but the presence of a dehydrated disc which coincides with the level of clinical midline deep tenderness is usually indicative. This underlines the importance of a detailed clinical examination. If there is a dehydrated disc at L.4/5 with clinical tenderness only at L5/S1 then I would advise a two level Graf stabilisation as 90% of low back problems occur at the lower two levels. Similarly, if there is clinical tenderness at L4/5 with a dehydrated disc at L4/5 and L5/S1, then I would also instrument both levels. If there is clinical tenderness and dehydration only at the L.4/5 level, then there is an argument for not instrumenting the L5/S1 disc, especially in a young patient. Similarly, a non-tender MRI normal L4/5 disc is usually not instrumented in younger patients with symptoms and dehydration at L5/S1.

Having started four years ago by trying to be very scientific and instrumenting only demonstrably symptomatic discs, I have had to stabilise additional MRI abnormal levels in a small number of patients and am therefore inclined to stabilise dehydrated discs at the lower three levels. If MRI scanning reveals multi-level lumbar disc disease, then the levels of clinical tenderness are certainly important and discography is often helpful in determining which are the symptomatic discs. There should be no hesitation in carrying out a three level instrumentation as, unlike spinal fusion surgery, three level instrumentations seem to do just as well as one or two levels, provided the correct levels are stabilised.

I have done one 5 level and three 4 level instrumentations for multi-level disc disease with worthwhile results but always as an add-on around a year after the initial three level surgery because of symptoms in the higher discs. By that time some movement has returned in the lower discs, making stabilisation of the additional levels less restrictive.

Provocative discography is of practical clinical use in those patients in whom there is uncertainty as to the level of the pain source. Discography can only indicate a discogenic pain source and it is invasive and often painful but it gives, at least in my experience, clinically useful information in around 80% of patients on whom the investigation is performed. Since discography is painful and there is also a small incidence of infection, I believe it should be performed selectively. Discography cannot reproduce posterior column symptoms which probably accounts for the 20% unreliability factor with this investigation.

MRI scanning may indicate a normal spine in highly symptomatic patients, especially those under thirty years old. In those patients with apparently genuine symptoms, discography may be the only way of identifying the symptomatic level and is most useful in this respect[13].

6. The Graf technique

The system comprises titanium pedicular screws placed above and below the symptomatic disc and connected by longitudinal bands (Figure 7). The screws have a cancellous thread with a shaft diameter of 5, 6 or 7 mm. The available lengths are 35, 40 and 45 mm. The screws have a conical section above the thread with a sintered surface. The tops of the screws have a hemispherical flange which retains the bands securely in position. Middle pedicular screws for instrumentation of two or more levels are available in the same sizes with a longer outer section to accommodate two bands which are retained in place by addition of a titanium screw cap.

Titanium protective sleeves (diabolos) may also be used to protect the bands from abrasion by the facet joints. In practice these are unnecessary as this problem can be avoided by removal with an osteotome of any part of the facet joint in contact with the band. This is an important precaution. A diabolo may also be useful occasionally to tension a band if it is felt to be a little loose.

The bands are made of braided polyester (Dacrilene™), the length varies with 2.5 mm increments from 15 to 50 mm and by 5 mm increments up to 75 mm. Bands over 35 mm are rarely required. Sizes 17.5 to 25 mm are the most commonly used. A radio-opaque marker is incorporated into the band.

Double thickness bands have been available since 1993 and have been clinically evaluated by Dr. Graf and others. These stronger bands appear to have some advantage over the single bands in use previously when used in tall or heavy patients. Sometimes such patients have seemed to undergo some degree of deterioration in their good results after 3 to 6 months which may be prevented by using the stronger bands (Figure 8).

A thorough programme of *in-vitro* testing has been undertaken by the manufacturer Safir and the bands and screws have now reached a design state where mechanical failure is a rarity[26]. The shaft/thread junction of the pedicle screws was strengthened in 1991 and, in my experience, this has completely eliminated the occasional screw breakage which occurred previously. I have identified only one band breakage in a series of over 300 cases. This was probably caused by chafing against the facet joint. It is crucial to ensure that the stitched join of the band is placed laterally away from the facet joint and also that no part of the band is touching bone. If there is any bone impingement then that piece of bone should be removed with a 5 mm osteotome.

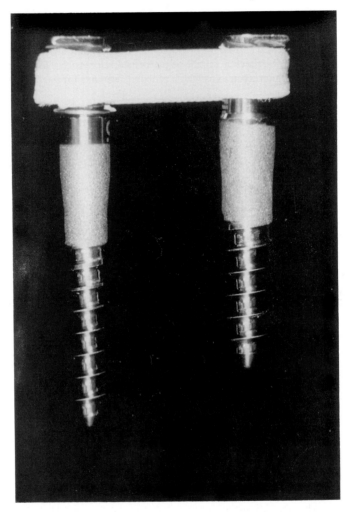

Figure 7. The titanium screws and Dacrilene band are shown. The conical sintered shaft of the pedicle screw engages firmly in the bone and provides excellent sheer strength as well as pull-out strength. The Dacrilene bands stretch by approximately 20% during the first 4-6 months allowing some return of movement to the motion segment and relieving the screws and bands of all but intermittent stresses. Screw and band breakage is therefore rare (less than 1%)

7. Results

A prospective study of the first 50 consecutive patients on whom I carried out Graf stabilisation was undertaken[12]. These patients were independently reviewed on average

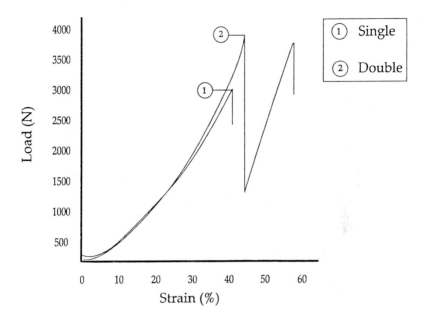

Figure 8(a). Load-deformation curves for single and double 25 mm bands. Double bands are about 20% stronger than single bands. They have similar stretch characteristics. It is likely that they stretch by 10% or 15% during the first week as the rectangular weave of the bands accommodates to the imposed stresses. A further gradual relaxation of 10% to 15% is then thought to occur over the next 3 to 6 months allowing some movement to return.

two years post-operatively and all were seen personally by Michael Grevitt, a Spinal Fellow from the unit of Professor Robert Mulholland of the University of Nottingham. I took no part in the review of these patients, nor in the analysis of the figures. The mean follow-up period was 24 ± 4 months (mean ± SD).

All patients underwent Oswestry Disability[5] scoring and the level of distress was assessed by means of the modified somatic perception questionnaire (MSPQ) and the Zung depression index[23]. The MSPQ and Zung questionnaires form part of the Distress and Risk Assessment Method (DRAM). DRAM may be used to predict the likely outcome of treatment[19]. One patient was involved in litigation at the time of surgery. The DRAM category was applied retrospectively to this series and therefore the surgical decisions were not influenced by it. The decision to operate was made on clinical grounds, supported by identification of a painful motion segment, by MRI or discography.

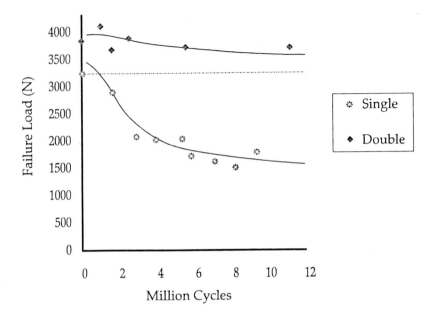

Figure 8(b). Mean failure load of 25 mm bands after fatigue testing at 500 N and 5 Hz. The superior performance of the double bands after cyclical loading is evident. In fact, it seems unlikely that heavy loading will occur *in vitro* after the first 3 months as a result of band stretching and a variable degree of disc narrowing which both result in de-tensioning of the bands.

Patients were classified as:

a) excellent, i.e. leading a normal life with no restrictions in sporting or social life.
b) good involved minor restrictions with intermittent non-disabling pain and a substantially normal lifestyle.
c) fair indicated a definite post-operative improvement but with a significant disability continuing and pain causing some disability at times.
d) the same meant no significant change in disability or level of symptoms
e) worse experienced a deterioration in their function with an increase in their symptoms compared with the pre-operative state.

The clinical result was:

excellent	17 (34%)
good	19 (38%)
fair	5 (10%)
the same	8 (16%)
worse	1 (2%)

Three patients regretted having surgery although one was classified as a good outcome.

Of those that returned to work, 27 (54%) did so within three months. 32 patients (64%) returned fulltime to their former occupation, 3 had a part time job and 8 patients remained unemployed at a time of relatively severe economic recession. The remainder were either housewives or those who took early retirement.

The mean pre-operative Oswestry Disability score was 59% (SD ±10%). At review the Disability level had decreased to 31% (SD ±9%) (Figure 9). The mean pre-operative Disability scores for the various groups were:

excellent	54 (SD ±22)
good	62 (SD ±16)
fair	58 (SD ±20)
the same	62 (SD ±10)
worse	78 (one patient)

Post-operatively the scores changed to:

excellent	18 (SD ±15)
good	30 (SD ±12)
fair	51 (SD ±11)
the same	50 (SD ±11)
worse	53

The excellent/good results (Group A) were compared to the fair/same/worse group (Group B). There was no significant difference between the groups in terms of age, duration of symptoms or pre-operative disability score. However, the post-operative disability scores were significantly different for Group A (24 ± 14) and Group B (51 ± 11) [$P < 0.01$, Student's t-test]. There was no difference in the post-operative lordosis angle, nor the change in angle in the flexion/extension views at the latest follow-up (Chi-squared test).

8. Complications

There were 27 complications, mostly of a minor nature, in 17 patients. There were no thrombo-embolic complications.

The commonest complication was post-operative radicular pain that was not present prior to surgery. The majority had minor symptoms that settled with symptomatic treatment. In 4 cases there was a persistent neurological deficit with some weakness of dorsiflexion in one patient and some quadriceps weakness in another. The other two had sensory disturbance only. Both these patients were pleased with the improvement in their back pain.

There were 3 screw breakages (1.2% of screws used) in 2 patients. These occurred at 12 and 18 months after surgery. This complication has not occurred since 1991 when the screw thread junction was strengthened.

DISABILITY SCORES

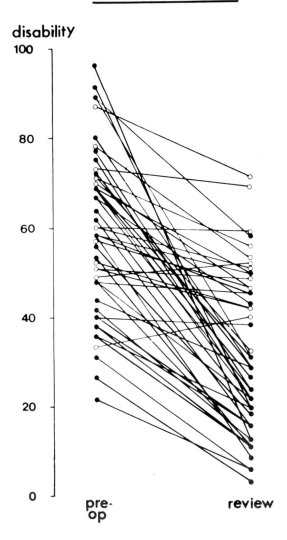

Figure 9. Oswestry Disability scores. 50 patients were independently reviewed on average 24 months post-operatively (range 19-36 months). White circles - male, black circles - female. In this series there was no radiological predictor of clinical outcome. Age, duration and level of disability were also random factors. A larger series may indicate discriminating factors.

Subsequent experience with over 300 cases has resulted in no acute infection but a late infection rate six months or more after surgery of around 2%. In all patients, removal of the implant has so far not compromised the pain relief they experienced with the original surgery. This lends weight to the theory that the Graf implant has its major effect during the first six months in allowing the symptomatic disc to stabilise. Presumably, after six months, the Graf implant stays in place as a checking band which may act to prevent the recurrence of hypermobility following excessive strains on the back which may occur from time to time.

The fact that band and screw breakage is so unusual indicates that there is probably no continuing stress on the implant after the first six months, firstly because the bands have stretched by 20% to 30%, as indicated in *in vitro* studies and secondly, because the disc has narrowed to some extent as a result of the compression force applied by the Graf implant and through the natural history of disc degeneration. This narrowing will, of course, bring the pedicle screws closer together further reducing the tension in the band.

Two patients underwent revision operations following sudden recurrence of symptoms 4 and 16 weeks after surgery. The radio opaque markers in the bands were noted to be broken and ruptured bands were suspected. At exploration the bands were intact but smaller bands were required to re-establish stability and a good clinical result. All the patients in this series were stabilised with single thickness bands. It is expected that double thickness bands, available since 1993, will eliminate this problem. Subsequent experience has shown that the radio opaque markers sometimes rupture after 4 to 6 months but this is of no clinical significance as they are clearly less elastic than the bands themselves.

Four patients who gained no pain relief after Graf stabilisation underwent repeat discography which provoked the same pain that they had had before surgery and anterior fusion was carried out. None achieved better than a fair result.

9. Conclusions

The above series[12] relates to the first 50 patients operated on by the author and contained inevitable learning curve errors. However, the results were sufficiently encouraging to continue Graf stabilisation for patients suffering from intolerable symptoms from degenerative disc disease as these results were considered to be as good as, if not better than, those obtained by spinal fusion for this condition.

Graf stabilisation has some further advantages over spinal fusion:

1. The operation appears to be more physiological. It allows some movement to return to the stabilised motion segment which is likely to encourage better neuromuscular activity and reduce stress on adjacent discs.

2. The operation is less invasive with limited dissection around the facet joints and therefore less muscle denervation, with a quicker recovery of lumbar muscle function.

3. Since there is no bone grafting, rehabilitation can be comparatively rapid with most patients returning to work after 10 or 12 weeks. Hospitalisation time of 5 to 8 days is also reduced compared with spinal fusion.

4. Since there is no bone grafting, there is no risk of pseudoarthrosis and no donor site pain. The results do not appear to deteriorate with the number of levels instrumented; it is only important that the correct levels are instrumented.

5. The operation is substantially quicker than an instrumented spinal fusion and therefore cheaper. It is also less exhausting for the surgeon. With practise, a single level Graf instrumentation can be carried out in one hour and 3 levels in two hours.

The disadvantages of Graf instrumentation are:

1. Immobilisation of the motion segment in extension may result in radicular pain. If there is any significant disc narrowing, hypermobility (especially in extension), or any clinical suspicion of pre-operative radicular pain, then either discectomy and/or foraminal decompression by flavectomy and/or undercutting facetectomy should be carried out, followed by probing to make sure that the foramen and the lateral recess are clear.

2. There appears to be a risk of late blood-born infection (approximately 2%). If this occurs, removal of the entire implant is necessary but, fortunately, this does not seem to compromise the final clinical result.

3. The Graf implant is relatively expensive with prices approximating to those of the more expensive pedicle screw fusion systems.

It seems reasonable to conclude that Graf flexible stabilisation represents a desirable alternative to stabilisation by instrumented or non-instrumented fusion in degenerative disc disease. This operation should not be undertaken by surgeons inexperienced in the implantation of pedicle screws[9] and it is essential that the symptomatic motion segment is positively identified so far as is possible.

Extensive clinical study of the Graf stabilisation technique appears to be justified and those wishing to undertake the procedure should carry out prospective physical and psychological disability assessments so that objective outcomes can be reported.

Surgeons undertaking the Graf procedure are recommended to take part in the International Outcome Study being co-ordinated by Dr. Guy Declerck of Aalst, Belgium, from whom clinical study pro formas can be obtained (Fax No. 010 32 53 786521)

10. Acknowledgements

My thanks are due to Mrs. Sylvia Bennett who typed and revised the drafts of this paper.

11. References

1. N. Bogduk, W. Tynan and A.S. Wilson, *J. Anat.* **132** 39.
2. S.P. Chow, J.C.Y. Leong, A. Ma and A.C.M.C. Yau, *Spine* **5** (1980) 452.
3. R.B. Cloward, *Clin. Orthop.* **193** (1985) 16.
4. M.A. Edgar and J.A. Ghadially, *Clin. Orthop.* **115** (1976) 35.
5. J.C.T. Fairbank, J. Couper, J.B. Davies and J.P. O'Brien, *Physiotherapy* **66** (1980) 271.
6. J.C.T. Fairbank, W.M. Park, I.W. McCall and J.P. O'Brien, *Spine* **6** (1981) 598.
7. H.F. Farfan and W.H. Kirkaldy-Willis, *Clin. Orthop.* **158** (1981) 198.
8. D. Freebody, R. Bendall and R.D. Taylor. *J. Bone Joint Surg.* **53-B** (1971) 617.
9   S.R. Garfin, *et al.*, *Spine* **19** (1994) 20S.
10. H. Graf, *Rachis* **4** (1992) 123.
11. H. Graf, personal communication 1989.
12. M.P. Grevitt, A.D.H. Gardner, J. Spilsbury, I.M. Shackleford, R. Baskeville, L.M. Purcell, A. Hassaan and R.C. Mulholland, The Graf stabilisation system: early results in 50 patients. *Eur. Spine J.* (1994 in press)
13. A.E. Heilman and J.P. O'Brien, *J. Bone Joint Surg.* **72-B** (1990) 1088.
14. V.T. Inman and J.B. De L. Saunders, *J. Nervous & Mental Disorders* **99** (1944) 660.
15. J.H. Kellgren, The anatomical source of back pain. *Rheumatol. & Rehabilitation* XVI(1) 7.
16. W.H. Kirkaldy-Willis and H.F. Farfan, *Clin. Orthop.* **165** (1982) 110.
17. J.A. Kozak and J.P. O'Brien, *Spine* **15** (1990) 322.
18. S.D. Kuslich, C.L. Ulstrom and C.J. Michael, *Orthop. Clinics of N. America* **22** (1991) 2.
19. C.J. Main and G. Waddell, *Spine* **17** (1992) 42.
20. D.S. McNally and M.A. Adams, *Spine* **17** (1991) 66.
21. J.P. O'Brien and D.C. Holte, *Eur. Spine J.* **1** (1992) 2.
22. S. Olerud, L. Sostrum, G. Karlstrom and M. Hamburg, *Clin. Orthop.* **203** (1986) 67.
23. P. Pynsent, J.C.T. Fairbank and A. Carr, *Outcome Measures in Orthopaedics*, (Butterworth & Heinemann, 1993) pp 108-143.
24. S. Rolander, *Acta Orthop. Scand.* **90** (1966) 1.
25. S. Sacks, *Orth. Clin. N. America* **6** (1975) 275.
26. SAFIR, 81 Avenue de la Republique, 92120 Montrouge, Paris, France. Fax 33(1)40 84 82 58
27. D.J. Selby, R.J. Henderson, in *The Adult Spine*, ed. J.W. Frymoyer, (Raven Press, New York) pp 1989-2006.
28. J.A.N. Shepperd, Spinal probing in the identification of pain sources in the low back. (personal communication)

29.   J. Soini and S. Seitsalo, Disc space heights after external fixation and
       anterior interbody fusion: a prospective 2 year follow-up of clinical and
       radiological results. ISSLS proceedings, Marseilles, France 1993
30.   A.D. Steffee, R.S. Biscup and D.J. Sitowski, *Clin. Orthop.* **203** (1986) 45.
31.   J.A. Turner, M. Ersek, L. Herron, J. Haselkorn, D. Kent, M.A. Ciol and
       R. Deyo, *J.A.M.A.* **268** (1992) 907.
32.   H. Vanharanta, B.L. Sachs, M.A. Spivey, R.D. Guyer, S.H. Hochschuler,
       R.F. Rashbaum, R.G. Johnson, D. Ohnmeiss and V. Mooney, *Spine* **12**
       (1987) 287.
33.   C.R. Weatherley, C.F. Prickett and J.P. O'Brien, *J. Bone Joint Surg.* **68-B**
       (1986) 142.
34.   A.A. White and M.M. Panjabi, *Clinical biomechanics of the spine* 2nd edn.,
       (J.B.Lippincott, Philadephia, 1990)
35.   L.L. Wiltse, *Clin. Orthop.* **35** (1964) 116.
36.   H. Yoshizawa, J.P. O'Brien, W.T. Smith and M. Trumper, *J. Pathology*
       132 (1980) 95.

CHAPTER 20

RADICAL RESECTION OF VERTEBRAL BODY TUMOURS: A SURGICAL TECHNIQUE USED IN TEN CASES

M.W. Fidler

1. Introduction

An operation for radical resection of a tumour of the vertebral body and part of the neural arch is described. The approach is posterior and from both sides of the spine.

The posterior approach is used to remove the healthy part of the neural arch, mobilise the dura, divide involved nerve roots and carry out the postero-lateral parts of the spinal osteotomies or disc divisions. On one side, usually the right, the sides of the vertebral body or bodies are freed and the osteotomies or disc divisions are extended. Then from the other side, a posterolateral thoracotomy or lumbotomy allows completion of the dissection with radical resection by rolling the specimen away from the dura.

Ten operations are reported in which up to three and a half vertebrae were resected. Spinal reconstruction was by internal fixation and grafting preferably with vascularised bone. The results were satisfactory after follow-up for as long as eight years.

In 1985, a patient presented for further surgical treatment of a giant-cell tumour of an upper thoracic vertebral body which had spread into the apex of the left lung (case 1, Figure 1). After full investigation, a combined posterior and bilateral anterolateral approach was used to resect the whole of the tumour mass *en-bloc*. This type of operation has now been used in ten patients to achieve radical or nearly radical resection of extensive tumours of the vertebral body. The basic principles of the radical resection have not changed, but improved techniques of stabilisation and reconstruction have been developed.

The present technique and its complications and possible pitfalls are described and discussed.

2. Pre-operative investigation and planning

Routine investigations include radiography, bone scans and CT. MRI has supplanted CT myelography; it delineates the tumour, shows dural compression and is particularly useful for assessing the neighbouring vertebrae and for showing local soft-tissue extension of the tumour. Biopsy, selective angiography and, when appropriate, embolisation are carried out; these are discussed later.

2.1 Antibiotics
Cephamandole (2 g) is injected intravenously before surgery and repeated 6-hourly for 48 hours. At present, we use pre-operative selective intestinal sterilisation[21].

2.2 Planning

Detailed planning is essential; each operation must be tailored as an individual resection. Schematic drawings based on the radiographs and the transverse MRI or CT scans are made (Figure 2). Using a skeleton for referral, the sites of division of the neural arch and the vertebral column are marked on the drawings. All bone and all soft tissue shown by MRI to be involved are included in the resection which is through a disc only if it is certain that the vertebral end plate is intact. If there is any doubt, resection is by osteotomy through the neighbouring healthy vertebral body.

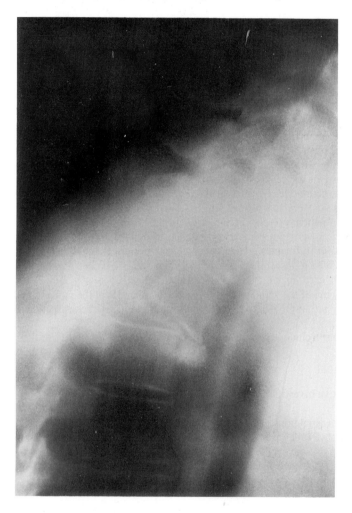

Figure 1. Case 1: Lateral tomogram (contd.)

It is easier to mobilise the aorta and divide the segmental vessels supplying the tumour from the left side. When possible, the left side is therefore chosen for the more major approach and removal of the tumour. If the tumour extends into the right half of the vertebral arch, right-sided removal will be required and in such a case, the aorta can usually be mobilised from the right during the final stage of the operation (case 4). If MRI shows that a mainly right-sided tumour completely obscures the aorta (cases 5 and 8; Figure 3), it is necessary to use a preliminary left-sided approach, with the patient lying on the right side, to mobilise the aorta from the tumour before repositioning for the final right-sided approach and tumour removal.

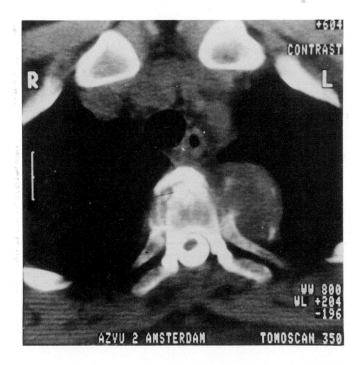

Figure 1 (Case 1 contd.). CT myelogram of a giant cell tumour arising from and causing collapse of the body of T3.

The blood supply of the spinal cord[4] is respected at all times. It is known that any number of segmental arteries may be divided unilaterally[11], but the dangers of bilateral division are unknown and are kept to a minimum.

When an uninvolved nerve root is to be spared, the posterior wall of its intervertebral foramen must be widely opened. If this would endanger the radical nature of the resection, then the nerve root must be sacrificed.

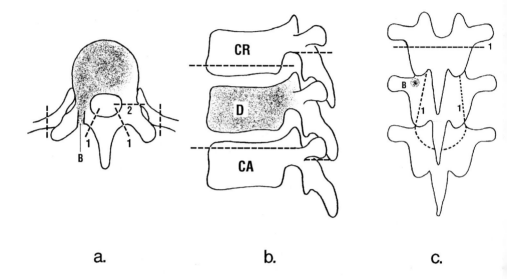

a.   b.   c.

Figure 2 a,b,c. Diagrams of the planned resection of a predominantly left-sided tumour. The laminae are initially removed along dashed lines '1'. The uninvolved transverse process and posterior part of the pedicle are removed up to dashed line '2'. B is the site of a previous open transpedicular biopsy. D is the involved vertebra. If more vertebrae are involved, D is the most cranial involved vertebra. CR is the adjacent cranial vertebra. CA is the adjacent caudal vertebra.

In addition to drawings, it is helpful to write an *aide-memoire* of the various steps of the planned operation.

3. Surgical technique

This is described for a predominantly left sided tumour of the thoracic spine (Figure 2). A similar technique is used for more caudal tumours but release of the diaphragm and/or psoas is also required.

3.1 Stage one

The patient is placed prone, with facilities for biplanar image intensification, and, if necessary, the spinal level is checked radiologically. A midline incision is used to expose the spine to the tips of the transverse processes (Figure 4). Any biopsy or previous operation scar is excised and the edges examined by frozen section. When a previous open transpedicular biopsy has been carried out, the hole in the pedicle is identified to confirm the spinal level; this hole must be resected with the specimen. The planned spinous processes, laminae and inferior facets (Figure 2) are removed with a small oscillating saw[7] or punches. When a lamina has been penetrated by tumour (case 8) it is left in the resection block with a thin covering of muscle. If division through a disc is planned, access is obtained by removing the superior articular processes of the diseased vertebra (D, Figure 2b); if an articular process is involved and cannot be removed, osteotomy is required through the body of the adjacent vertebra. The structures within the resection lines shown on Figure 2b are removed sequentially: the superior articular processes of the caudal vertebra (CA), the uninvolved part of the right pedicle and transverse process of the diseased vertebra (D), the medial end of the right rib of vertebra D. The left rib of vertebra D is then divided just lateral to the tip of the transverse process.

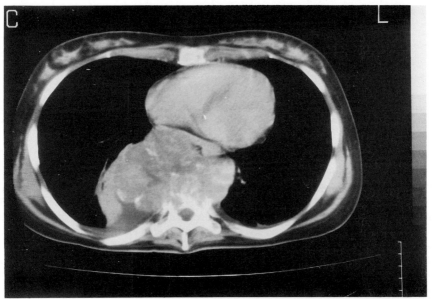

Figure 3. Case 5: MRI shows the aorta displaced to the left by a large midthoracic giant-cell tumour. This was removed through a right thoracotomy after mobilising the aorta through a left thoracotomy.

Any nerve roots which are involved by the tumour, or which will prevent the involved block resection being rolled out, are tied close to the dura and divided. At a later stage, they are sectioned beyond the tumour.

The dura is mobilised to just beyond the levels of the planned osteotomies or disc divisions and gently elevated with soft rubber bands. The epidural veins are coagulated with bipolar diathermy and divided. Large anterolateral epidural veins are better ligated.

Holes for the pedicle screws for reconstruction are made in the routine manner[2], with the extra safeguard that the entrance points are first marked with the points of Kirschner wires and their positions checked by image intensifier. The sites for the spinal osteotomies or disc divisions are verified at the same time. Above T6, if the pedicles are small, laminar wires or claw-hook systems are used instead of screws.

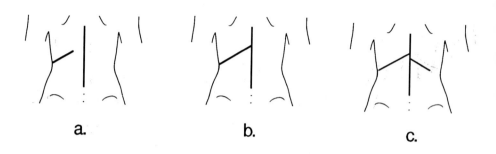

a.   **b.**   **c.**

Figure 4. Skin incisions. a) Suitable for a thin patient. The view of the tumour during the second stage is impaired by the musculocutaneous bridge, but wound closure is easy. b) The usual incision. c) Applicable when extra exposure is required.

3.2 Lateral release of the tumour

The right side of the spine is exposed extrapleurally through the midline incision by excising the posterior 2 cm of the rib of vertebra D, and of vertebra CA if necessary, and elevating the pleura with a finger or small pledget. This dissection is more difficult if the transverse process is involved and has to be left in situ until excised *en bloc*. If possible, segmental vessels are elevated from the side of the vertebral body and spared. If the tumour has broken through the cortex on the right side, then the pleura is not elevated, but divided around the tumour. In this instance better exposure is obtained by a short posterolateral thoracotomy above the rib of vertebra D, using an additional oblique skin incision (see Figure 4c) with the patient still in a prone position.

The posterolateral parts of the spinal osteotomies or disc divisions are now performed. The posterior longitudinal ligament and the underlying bone or annulus can usually be divided at this stage, gaining access by retracting the dura gently first to one side and then the other. If undue dural retraction would be required to reach the midline, this stage is left until later when these midline structures can be approached from the side during removal of the diseased vertebral segment. The appropriate costotransverse ligaments are divided, and the osteotomies are extended anteriorly on the right side, with gently retraction of the soft tissues. The pedicle holes are tapped and on the right side the screws are inserted and a contoured plate is secured. On the left side, the screws holes are marked with pieces of a catheter. The wound is closed.

3.3 Stage two

The patient is repositioned for the second stage, at once or after an overnight stay in the intensive care unit.

A posterolateral left-sided thoracotomy is made above the rib of vertebra D or, in the lower thoracic spine, above the rib of vertebra CR. Lesions involving the upper four thoracic vertebrae (cases 1 and 7) are approached through the bed of, or above, the third rib after the scapula has been mobilized by releasing its muscular attachments from the spinous processes[11]. Osteotomies of the angles of the adjacent ribs improve exposure. The erector spinae muscles are divided transversely and turned down with a triangular skin flap to beyond the tumour. The posterior edge of the diaphragm is released if necessary (cases 2, 4 and 8). The pleura is incised along the sulcus between the aorta and the vertebral body, or more anteriorly if necessary, and then transversely over the spine at the sites of the planned osteotomies or disc deivisions. The sympathetic trunk is mobilised forwards if possible; otherwise it is divided. The splanchnic nerves are spared where possible. The aorta is mobilised forwards by dividing the segmental vessels as necessary. If possible, the stumps of an artery and one vein are left long to facilitate subsequent anastomosis with the vessels of the bone graft.

The posterior wound is reopened and irrigated. To make certain that the vertebrae are free, fingers are passed lateral to the plate, round the right side of the spine to emerge behind the aorta. With the dura clearly visible, the osteotomies or disc divisions are completed, and the anterior longitudinal ligament is divided. The plate is then loosened at one end to allow the osteotomies or disc divisions to open slightly and the involved vertebra(e) are rolled out laterally and forwards with the dura still under direct vision. Any remaining epidural veins require bipolar coagulation and are divided with any remaining soft tissue connection. Any suspect tissue at the edge of the resection is biopsied and sent for frozen section. The wound is copiously rinsed with Dakin's solution followed by saline.

3.4 Stabilisation

The pedicle screws on the left side are inserted in the marked holes and a contoured plate is loosely attached. Depending on their thickness and the size of the spine, one or two tricortical iliac-crest grafts, one of them preferably vascularized, are inserted anteriorly and clamped in place as the pedicle screw nuts are tightened. The vascular anastomosis is carried out. Cancellous chips are added anteriorly and corticocancellous strips are placed posterolaterally (Figure 5).

The iliac crest is reconstituted with either part of a rib or a small AO plate and bone slivers. The wound is closed over appropriate drains.

3.5 Postoperative management

Provided that sound pedicle screw and plate stabilisation have been combined with a secure, good-quality anterior graft, the patient is mobilised as soon as possible in a brace appropriate to the level of the operation. If there is any doubt about the quality of the reconstruction the patient should is kept in bed until the graft incorporates; this is a major curative operation and the risks msut be kept to a minimum.

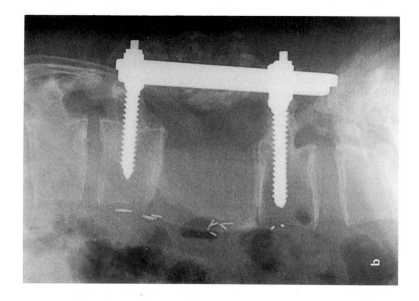

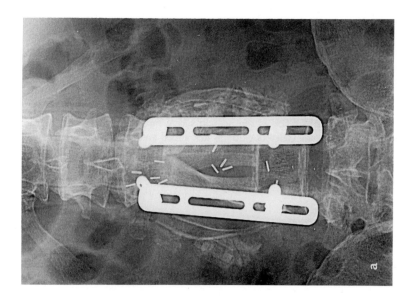

Figure 5. Case 3: a) Anteroposterior and b) lateral radiographs after resection of L3 for chordoma and stabilisation of the spine.

3.6 Case reports including problems and complications

These are summarized in Tables 1 and 2. Furthermore there was severe epidural bleeding in cases 5 and 8. In case 5 the second stage of the operation had to be postponed for two weeks when further severe bleeding precluded the insertion of a time-consuming vascularised graft. In case 8 the insertion of a vascularised graft had to be delayed for two weeks, temporary anterior stabilisation being achieved with a modern version of the tumour jack previously described[6].

4. Discussion

Radical resection of vertebral bodies by a purely posterior approach has been reported[15,18-20]. This has the advantage that the patient does not need repositioning for a posterolateral thoracotomy, but the total extent of the dissection, more on one side and less on the other, is similar to the present technique. The purely posterior technique is applicable when the lesion is limited to the vertebral body and the neighbouring soft tissues can be easily and safely stripped from the bone. This was not possible in some of the reported cases because of lung involvement (case 1), extensive adhesions after previous operations (cases 6, 9 and 10), a paravertebral fracture haematoma (case 2), or because of the diffulty of mobilizing and delivering a large tumour through a posterior wound (cases 5 and 8). In these circumstances the present technique appears to have an advantage. It enables radical resection of all involved tissue under direct vision and allows unhindered access to, and control of, the blood supply to the tumour.

Successful radical resection has two prerequisites. First, part of the vertebral arch and the underlying epidural space must be normal so that the bony ring around the dura can be broached through healthy tissue and allow the diseased vertebral segment to be rolled away from the dural tube. Secondly, it must be possible to divide any involved nerve root at its junction with the dura without overhanging tumour leading to possible contamination of the operation site (this occurred in cases 7 and 8). Radical excision after a previous intralesional excision must always be suspect, but the operation seems to be worthwhile for giant-cell tumours (cases 1 and 6).

A similar operation, combining posterior approach with a thoracotomy, reported by Larssen[13], but in this case intralesional excision of the grade-III giant-cell tumour was unavoidable; the operation was successful. Krajbich and Eldridge[12] also reported a similar technique, but they routinely sacrificed the nerve roots bilaterally at the level of the lesion; this is not always necessary. Their three patients all had a spinal metastasis from an osteosarcoma, and their longest follow-up was three years. Weinstein[23] also described the concept of combined anterior and posterior approaches, but the 'osteotomies' would transgress tumour extending from the body into the pedicle. This techniqe has now been modified (personal communication).

The improvement in techniques of spinal stabilisation has facilitated the development of the operation. In the first two patients, a Hartshill rectangle was used for posterior stabilisation. The rectangle should normally be wired to two vertebrae above and two below the lesion to give rigid fixation, but this would have prevented subsequent correction of the kyphotic deformity unless it was temporarily removed and reshaped,

Table 1: Details of ten patients having radical resection of vertebral body tumour

Case	Age (Yr)	Sex	Presentation	Diagnosis
1	34	F	Progressive destruction of T3 Ingrowth to left lung Laminectomy T2, T3, T4 T5, partial tumour resection, 45 Gy, 8 months previously	Giant-cell I
2	27	M	Backpain Pathological fracture T12 Destruction of T12 + pedicles	Posterolateral percutaneous biopsy Giant-cell I
3a	48	M	Backpain Destruction of L3 + pedicles, L>R	Posterolateral percutaneous biopsy Chordoma
b			2 years later, increasing pain	Broken screws, graft collapse
4	26	F	Pain Tumour, body and R pedicle T12 Referred after percutaneous biopsy	Giant-cell III
5	27	F	Pain Tumour in T7, T8, T9 + large anterior + R paravertebral extension on to T5, T6 and T10	Open transpedicular biopsy right Giant-cell I
6a	22	F	Painful collapse of T9, Paraparesis Tumour in T7, T8 and T9 + left lamina T9 Partial resection 4 years previously	Broken screws, graft fracture
b			1.5 years later, severe paraparesis	Giant-celll III
7	28	F	Left paravertebral tumour progression, 11 months after cord compression Laminectomy T1-T2, partial tumour removal, 50, 4 Gy	Solitary metastasis Phaeochromocytoma removed 16 years previously
8	29	M	Tumour T11 Paravertebral extension R sides of T10 and 12, lamina T11 right Previous biopsy	Giant-cell Biopsy II Specimen III
9	33	M	Control bone scan Tumour T7	Right open transpedicular biopsy: osteosarcoma-metastasis 1982. Left femur: resection of osteosarcoma and rotationplasy
10	17	M	Control Tumour T5, T6	Right open transpedicular biopsy: osteosarcoma-metastasis Resection of paraspinal osteosarcoma (right 5, 6, 7 ribs) 6 months previously

Table 2: Details of ten patients having radical resection of vertebral body tumour

Case	Resection*	Stabilisation	Postoperative management	Follow-up/result
1	T(2)T3T(4) Left 3rd rib	Rectangle T1-T6,T7 Non-vascularised graft	Bed 3 months Milwaukee 1 year	8 years No symptoms Moderate kyphosis
2	T12	Rectangle + anterior Zielke T11-L1	Bed 3 months Boston brace 1 year	8 years Occasional backache
3a	L3 Left lumbotomy	Steffee L2-L4 Non-vascularised graft	Boston brace 2 months postop, 56 Gy	5 years See 3b
3b		Steffee renewed Vascularised graft Multiple biopsies No tumour	Boston brace + crutches for 2 years	Graft solid Almost painfree Cycles 50 km/day
4	T(11),T12 Right 10th rib	Steffee T11-L1 Non-vascularised graft + pedicled rib graft	Boston brace 1 year	4 years No symptoms Metal removed after 3 years
5	T(6),T7,T8,T9 Tumour dissected off T5,T6,T10 Right 5th rib	Non-vascularised graft Anterior slot-Zielke Pedicle screws T10, Steffee plates, laminar wires T5	Bed 6 weeks High Boston brace 2 years	3 3/4 years Thoracic spine consolidated Painfree. Weak anterior abdominal muscles due to division of T7,T8,T9 roots bilaterally
6a	T7,T8,T9T(10) Left 6th rib	Steffee T6-11 Vascularised graft	Bed 3 months Milwaukee 2 years	3 1/4 years See 6b
6b		Series of 3 operations Cord decompression Restablisation:pedicle screws T11,T12 Isola rods, laminar wires T3,4,5 Wisconsin compression Anterior vascularised fibula graft T5 to T11 Multiple biopsies:no tumour	Bed 6 months Boston/Milwaukee brace	Good neurological recovery Graft consolidation
7	(1),T2,T(3) Left 3rd rib	Rectangle C6,C7-T3,T4 Non-vascularised graft	Halo cuirass 3 months	1 3/4 years Horner left, otherwise well
8	T(10),T11,T(12) Right 10th rib	Steffee T9,T10-T12(L),L1 Non-vascularised graft	Bed 3 months Boston brace 1 year	1 1/2 years Spine symptom-free Multiple lung metastases
9	T(6),T7,T(8) Right 7th rib	Steffee T6-T9 Vascularised graft	Milwaukee brace 50 Gy Chemotherapy (adriamycin, cisplatin)	1 1/4 years Well
10	T5,T6 Right 5th rib	CD Pedicle screws T7,T8 Laminar + pedicle hooks T2(R),T3 Vascularised graft	Milwaukee, 45 Gy Chemotherapy (CESS)	9 months Pulmonary metastases

vertebrae with numbers in parentheses were partially resected
thoracotomies were carried out above the rib mentioned except in case 1 in which the rib was excised
all patients had additional posterolateral autograft fusions

KEY TO TABLES
Gy   Radiotherapy: Gray
Vg   Anterior Vascularised iliac crest autograft.
NVg   Anterior Non-vasularized iliac crest autograft.
(All patients had additional postero-lateral chip iliac crest autograft fusions.)
        * RESECTION.
Vertebra with numbers in parentheses were partially resected.
Left/right refers to the side of the major operation.
Thoracotomies were carried out above the rib mentioned except in case 1 where the rib was excised.

with the associated dangers. Such an extensive fixation would also have unnecessarily extended the fused region of the spine. In case 1, concomitant anterior Zielke stabilisation made it possible to limit the rectangle fusion to two levels below and one level above the lesion and, in case 2, to one level above and one level below. In both cases, for added safety, the patients were nursed flat in bed for three months and protected by long-term bracing. The use of pedicle screws and plates[17] with anterior and posterolateral bone grafting usually allows safe, early mobilisation in an external brace (cases 3, 4 and 9). This remains the routine technique below midthoracic level where the pedicles are of sufficient size. Above this level laminar wiring (cases 1, 5 to 7) or claw-hook system (case 10) are more appropriate. Diagonal wiring or cross bridging prevents any 'windscreen wiper' effect. The posterior metal can be removed after bony consolidation to reduce the final stiffness of the fused segments, to avoid metal fatigue and to facilitate scanning in the event of a possible recurrence.

Safe, durable reconstruction of the spine depends on bone consolidation. Free autografts probably become incorporated at their ends within a few weeks, but complete revascularisation and remodelling can take a year or longer[3]. During this period, there is a risk of graft breakage or avascular necrosis. By contrast, vascularised grafts are usually rapidly incorporated. If a free vascularised graft from the iliac-crest is not technically possible, then a segment of rib on its vascular pedicle can be turned down to reinforce an anterior non-vascularised iliac-crest autograft (case 4). A free vascularised iliac-crest (or fibular) autograft is recommended when this is technically possible.

Radiotherapy may be indicated after operation (cases 3, 9 and 10). Radiotherapy delays fracture healing but rigid internal fixation mitigates this effect[1,9]. On the assumption that bone grafts would be similarly affected, radiotherapy in the present series was postponed for six weeks following operation; this is in keeping with the recent recommendation by Emery *et al.*[5].

Biopsy is essential before major tumour surgery. In six of the reported cases (1, 4, 6 to 8 and 10) the diagnosis had been made before referral. In case 3, the track of a posterolateral percutaneous biopsy was subsequently found to be contaminated and this had serious consequences. Similar contamination was possible in case 2. Open transpedicular biopsy[8] is now recommended when a primary resectable tumour is a possibility; the hole is blocked with bone wax. It is theoretically attractive to excise the open biopsy scar and track *en-bloc* with the diseased part of the vertebra, but in practice the ellipse of tissue containing the scar and track is an encumbrance. It is therefore cut from the bone specimen and examined histologically. To date, frozen sections of the tissue adjacent to the bone wax have been negative (cases 5, 9 and 10). The same procedure is followed for scar excision after a previous intralesional operation. Such excision can be beneficial; in case 1, histological examination showed giant-cell tumour tissue embedded in the excised scar.

Possible microscopic contamination at various stages has been mentioned. In each case, there was never any visible tumour spill and any area of possible contamination was widely resected with the specimen. MRI would have allowed better planning in case 2, and in case 4 the whole of the adjacent disc including the next vertebral end plate would now be included in the specimen. In cases 5, 7 and 8, the tumour had already grown to an unfavourable size and shape.

Preoperative selective angiography reveals the presence of any major medullary feeder artery[4], such as that of Adamkiewicz, or any vascular abnormalities near the tumour. If the tumour bed is hypervascular, it is embolized with Ivalon (Polystan Benelux, Almere Haven, The Netherlands), avoiding any segmental artery which gives rise to a major medullary feeder artery. Embolisation reduces the flow through the tumour into the epidural veins and minimises blood loss during the posterior part of the operation. During the transthoracic part of the operation the tumour is directly separated from its blood supply. Buds of tumour tissue may be present inside veins within the tumour (case 8), and prior reduction of blood flow may therefore reduce the risk of tumour dissemination during the operation.

Monitoring of the spinal cord was used only in case 5. This type of tumour surgery does not involve significant correction of deformity or cord distraction and the dura and any possible feeder arteries which accompany the nerve roots, are disturbed as little as possible. Cord monitoring during temporary clamping, however, may help in deciding how to deal with an artery which passes close to possible tumour tissue and which supplies a possibly important medullary feeder artery (case 10). In this case the operation would have been truly radical if it had been known that a doubtful blood vessel could have been sacrificed with impunity.

Radical resection can be a curative treatment for some spinal tumours. Sanjay *et al.*[16] recommended that "giant-cell tumours of the spine be completely removed but, because of their location, this usually means excision with an intralesional margin". The technique now described ensures complete removal of the tumour without the risk of recurrence associated with intralesional surgery. Local recurrences of giant-cell tumours take place within 2 years[10]. Pulmonary metastases occur in some 2% of cases and have been reported up to 10 years after resection of the primary tumour[14]. The disease-free period of eight years in cases 1 and 2 is encouraging, especially since in one patient the procedure was a reoperation and in the other a fracture with a paravertebral haematoma had already developed. Cases 4, 5 and 6 are disease-free at over three years. Radical resection is the only effective treatment for a chordoma[22]. Along with adjuvant chemotherapy and radiotherapy it is standard practice for osteosarcoma in the limbs and may be similarly applicable to the spine.

Extensive radical operations are time-consuming but improvements in anaesthesia and intensive care allow division into two stages. An uncomplicated operation can comfortably be performed by one spinal surgeon; the aid of a colleague to mobilise and anastomose the vascular pedicle of the iliac-crest graft provides a welcome break. For the complicated case, in which a large tumour is displacing or invading neighbouring structures, the early assistance of appropriately specialized surgical colleagues is beneficial.

5. Additional information and complications

5.1 Case 1
The excised posterior scar contained embedded giant cell tissue.

5.2 Case 2

Tumour encountered in the pedicles. No macroscopic contamination.

5.3 Case 3

Radiotherapy because a speck of tumour was found in the region of the biopsy track.

5.4 Case 4

During the final incision of the right side of the T11-T12 disc, tumour was encountered; immediate osteotomy above the inferior end plate of T11. No visible tumour contamination. The tumour had perforated the right side of the superior vertebral end-plate T12; this was not obvious on the MRI. Routine removal of metal, 3 years post-operatively.

5.5 Case 5

During posterior mobilization of the dura, severe epidural bleeding necessitated simple spinal stabilisation. Second stage postponed for 2 weeks. Severe bleeding during tumour removal; too ill for vascularized graft. Postero-lateral fusion added 6 weeks later. Two years later resection of sacral Giant Cell I tumour.

5.6 Case 6

Four years previously, partial resection of 'osteosarcoma' involving posterior ends of left 8 and 9 ribs and the sides of the vertebral bodies. Contaminated pleural cavity. Post-operative chemotherapy. Diagnosis revised prior to referral. At the time of the present resection, tumour was already in the spinal canal and had to be painstakingly separated from the dura. Macroscopically complete, though intralesional resection.
One and a half years later, broken screws T6, fractured graft, almost paraplegic. Series of 3 operations: posterior and anterior cord decompression. Partial correction of kyphosis. The postero-lateral 'fusion' consisted of dead bone chips in scar tissue. Restabilization with pedicle screws T11 and T12, Isola rods, laminar wires T3,T4,T5 and posterior Winsconsin compression system. Excision of the anterior pseudarthrosis. Anterior vascularised fibula graft T5-T11 and cancellous chips. Multiple biopsies: no recurrent tumour. Six months in bed. Mobilisation in Boston brace with Milwaukee extension. Neurological recovery. Graft consolidation.

5.7 Case 7

During the first stage of the resection it was necessary to elevate the edge of the tumour, which extended round the postero-lateral region of the epidural space, to reach and divide the involved left T1-T2 roots. During dissection through the epidural scar tissue, macroscopic tumour was not seen but routine frozen sections from the edge of the specimen were positive. The dura was further cleaned of all epidural tissue. At the beginning of the second stage, the nutrient artery arising from the costo-cervical trunk was divided from within the thorax.

5.8 Case 8

During the first stage of the operation a layer of muscle was left covering the biopsied lamina. During resection, the involved lamina and tumour had to be elevated to expose and divide the involved T11 nerve root: minimal tear in the capsule: no obvious tumour spill and local frozen sections were negative. Second stage: right thoracotomy above 10th rib: the aorta was too obscured by tumour for safe mobilization. One week later, aorta mobilized via left thoracotomy. One week later, right thoracotomy and posterior wounds re-opened, tumour removed. Oblique osteotomies through T10 and T12 to include the right sided paravertebral tumour extension. Revascularization of the anterior graft was unsuccessful. Three months in bed because of his heavy build and lack of vascularization of the graft. Boston brace and crutches for one year.

Histological examination of the specimen showed a giant cell tumour grade III with penetration into the lumina of many of the veins within the tumour. Six months later, numerous lung metastases discovered: too numerous for surgical resections or effective whole lung radiation.

5.9 Case 9

Similar lesions removed from left femur (rotationplasty 1982), right parietal bone (1986 and 1987), and left lung (July 1992). Fibrous nodule removed from right lung (July 1992). Following a left sided thoracotomy to free lung adhesions and mobilize the aorta, tumour removed through a right sided thoracotomy. Severe bloodloss. Temporary anterior tumour jack and cement[4,5]. Two weeks later, vascularized anterior iliac crest graft. Temporary tenderness over left proximal screw.

5.10 Case 10

Six months earlier, radical resection of osteosarcoma from posterior ends of left T5, T6 and T7 ribs. 'Solitary' meta-stasis in T5-T6. Vertebral resection: preliminary left thoracotomy to release scarring from the previous operation. Lung and aorta mobilized. Tumour removed through a right sided second stage. Attempt made to preserve the right 5th segmental artery which gave rise to a large medullary feeder artery. At the time it was felt unreasonable to possibly cause a paraplegia by the removal of a probably uninvolved artery, but frozen section of dubious tissue in the intervertebral foramen was positive. The vessel and adjacent tissue were therefore widely resected "en bloc". Apart from this possible but improbable microscopic contamination, the resection was radical.

All patients, except case 5, have either no or only minor symptoms due to division of segmental nerves.

6. Acknowledgements

I am most grateful to the various surgeons who have participated in some of the operations:
H. Been[†], K. Bloemendaal[*], L. Eysmans[*], J.Grünert[‡], H.Halm[†], A. Moulein[*], C. Plasmans[†], M. Sobotka[§], R. Soepaverta[*], P.Wuisman[†].
[*] cardiothoracic surgeon, [†] orthopaedic surgeon, [‡] plastic surgeon, [§] vascular surgeon

My thanks are due also to the anaesthetists and the intensive care specialists, in particular: Dr. C. Stoutenbeek, Dr. D. Zandstra and Dr. H. Oudemans.

5. References

1.   B.C. Bonarigo and P. Rubin, *Radiology* **88** (1967) 889.
2.   J.W. Brantigam, A.D. Steffee, L. Keppler, R.S. Biscup and P. Enker P, in *Spine: state of the art reviews* (Hanley & Belfus Inc, Philadelphia, 1992) 175.
3.   R.G. Burwell, in *Recent Advances in Orthopaedics*, ed. A.G. Apley, (J. & A. Churchill, London, 1969) 115.
4.   G.F. Dommisse, *Ann. R. Coll. Surg. Engl.* **62** (1980) 369.
5.   S.E. Emery, M.S. Brazinski, A. Koka and J.S. Bensusan, *J. Bone Joint Surg.* **76-A** 1994 540.
6.   M.W. Fidler, *J. Bone Joint Surg.* **68-B** (1986) 83.
7.   M.W. Fidler and E.B. Bongartz, *Spine* **13** (1988) 218.
8.   M.W. Fidler and B.B.A.M. Niers, *J. Bone Joint Surg.* **72-B** (1990) 884.
9.   B.J. Gainor and P. Buchert, *Clin. Orthop.* **178** (1983) 297.
10.   R.R. Goldenberg, C.J. Campbell and M. Bonfiglio, *J. Bone Joint Surg.* **52-A** (1970) 619.
11.   A.R. Hodgson, F.E. Stock, H.S.Y. Fang and G.B. Ong, *Br. J. Surg.* **48** (1960) 172.
12.   J.I. Krajbich and J. Eldridge, in *Complications of limb salvage: prevention, management and outcome*, ed. K.L.B. Brown (International Society of Limb Saving, Montreal, 1991) 391.
13.   S.E. Larsson, *J. Bone Joint Surg.* **61-B** (1979) 489.
14.   M.G. Rock, D.J. Pritchard and K.K. Unni, *J. Bone Joint Surg.* **66-A** (1984) 269.
15.   R. Roy-Camille, G. Saillant, M. Bisserié, Th. Judet, E. Hautefort and P. Mamoudy, *Revue de Chirurgie Orthopédique* **67** (1981) 421.
16.   B.K.S. Sanjay, F.H. Sim, K.K. Unni, R.A. McLeod and R.A. Klassen, *J. Bone Joint Surg.* **75B** (1993) 148.
17.   A.D. Steffee, R.S. Biscup and D.J. Sitkowski, *Clin. Orthop.* **203** (1986) 45.
18.   B. Stener, *J. Bone Joint Surg.* **53-B** (1971) 288-295.
19.   B. Stener, *Clin. Orthop.* **245** (1989) 72.
20.   B. Stener, O.E. Johnsen, *J. Bone Joint Surg.* **53-B** (1971) 278.
21.   C.P. Stoutenbeek, H.K. Van Saene, in *Host Defense Dysfunction in Trauma, Shock and Sepsis*, ed. E. Faist, J.L. Meakins, F.W. Schildberg (Springer-Verlag, Berlin, Heidelberg, 1993) 931.
22.   N. Sundaresan, Chordomas, *Clin. Orthop.* **204** (1986) 135.
23.   J.N. Weinstein, in *The adult spine. Principles and practice*, ed. J.W. Frymoyer (Raven Press Ltd., New York 1991) p.848.

CHAPTER 21

COSTS AND EFFECTIVENESS: APPROACHES TO THE MANAGEMENT OF BACK PAIN

J.A.K. Moffett and G. Richardson

1. Introduction

The costs of back pain to society are assumed to be high, and variably large figures are reported at intervals in the popular press, although they are not always based on reliable data or reasonable assumptions.

However, according to experts in the field, up to 85% of patients with back pain cannot be given a clear cut diagnosis[1-3]. The term non-specific mechanical low back pain is often used to categorise these patients, but perhaps should more appropriately be labelled as 'common low back pain'. The view that a strictly pathophysiological or mechanical approach to back pain is not effective, is emerging[4-7].

Frank (1993) noted that medical training may actually hinder a satisfactory therapeutic approach with an excessive emphasis on excluding serious although very uncommon pathology, rather than aiming to alleviate symptoms[8]. This may partly be related to a lack of training in this area, and also the limited amount of time that is spent on each consultation[9], which makes the appropriate provision of advice and health education difficult.

A study was recently carried out at the Centre for Health Economic (CHE) which provided estimates on the best available data on the uptake of health resources and other expenses related to back pain. The costs were divided into NHS, Local Authority, Out-of-pocket expenses and indirect costs.

2. NHS costs for back pain patients

Costs were estimated and adjusted where necessary for the UK population in 1992-93.

2.1. General practice

In order to estimate the costs of GP consultations for back pain a survey of 43 GPs in different areas of England was carried out by the Centre for Health Economics.[10] Five of the practices were based in the Birmingham area (with 29 GPs), one was in York (10 GPs) and another was in Exeter (with 4 GPs). In total they represented a population of 80,321 patients. The practices were selected primarily for their ability to provide reliable data. According to the results of this survey 6.4 % of the adult population consult their GP with back pain each year, which was in close agreement other studies[11,12]. The results also are consistent with data from other sources. For example the Intercontinental Medical Statistics (IMS) reported that 9.4% of the adult population have some contact with their general practice because of back pain each year. However, this is possibly an overestimate since it could include some repeat prescriptions for chronic or recurrent problems.

A rate of 2 consultations per annum was taken as the average for back pain. This was based on a rate of 1.5 from the CHE data, but balanced with a rate of 4 found by Coulter *et al.*[13] in their study of patients referred to out-patient clinics with back pain. The number of GP consultations for back pain in the UK was on this basis estimated to be in the range of 5.8 and 8.6 million resulting in a cost of £67.3 to £99.4 million, in 1992/93.

2.2. Prescriptions, GP referrals, radiology and physiotherapy

Data from the CHE survey[10], Papageorgiu survey[11], and IMS data were used to estimate numbers of prescriptions (mainly analgesics and NSAIDs), referrals to radiology, and referrals to out-patient clinics. Taken as a percentage of the total consultations for back pain these were respectively, 65% for prescriptions, 13% for radiology referrals, and 4.4-10.7 % for out-patient clinics referrals. The cost of physiotherapy was based on a survey carried out in Yorkshire and information from physiotherapists in Oxfordshire.[10] All these estimates are shown in Table 1.

2.3. Hospital in-patient admissions and day cases

According to data from the Hospital Episode Statistics[14], there were 897,000 bed days, 110,500 in-patients with dorsopathies (excluding trauma) in England, and approximately 40% of these were admitted for spinal surgery. It seems that more patients are being treated as day cases, but in 1989/90 (the most recent figures available)[14], these accounted for only a small proportion of the budget, as shown in Table 1.

Table 1. NHS Costs for Back Pain (1992/93 UK Figures)

NHS Category	Lower Estimate (£ million)	Upper Estimate (£ million)
General practice	67.3	99.4
Prescribed drugs	12.3	33.5
Out patients	11.6	55.6
Physiotherapy	24.0	36.0
Radiology	26.7	81.8
Day Cases	5.3	7.0
In-patients	117.4	122.4
TOTAL	**264.6**	**435.7**

3. Local authority expenses

Chronic back pain sufferers may use local authority services such as home helps, meals on wheels and social workers. According to the Office for Population Census's and Surveys (OPCS) 1985 Disability survey, this costs local government in the region of £23 million each year.

4. Out-of-pocket expenses

Out of pocket expenditure includes visits to private physiotherapists, osteopaths and chiropractors. Overall these consultations are estimated to be 4.5 million per annum, each costing approximately £20[10]. Based on information from IMS and the Proprietary Association of Great Britain[15], and assuming that 10-20 % of preparations bought over the counter, such as painkillers, are for back pain sufferers, these medications cost between £18 and £36 million per annum. There are many other out of pocket expenses incurred by people to ease their back pain, including "orthopaedic" mattresses, beds, chairs and even new cars, but the extent of this usage have not been quantified.

5. Indirect costs

Indirect costs consisting of productivity losses due individuals with back pain and their carers being absent from work, are high. Often Department of Social Security claims for certified days of sickness absence and invalidity benefits (503 million in 1991) have been cited as if they represented working days lost[*]. However, days of certified sickness include people who were not in the labour market, such as housewives. Also, these figures do not include people who are covered by Statutory Sickness Pay (SSP) or other employers' schemes. DSS claims have increased greatly over the past decade; 13.4% of claims in 1993 were for back pain. However in two independent large scale surveys, the total number of working days lost due to "sickness" for all causes was estimated to be between 168[16] and 200 million[17]. Assuming that back pain sufferers are representative of the general population in terms of salaries, an indirect cost of £1.2 to £1.7 billion for back pain is suggested.

There are other intangible costs which are even more difficult to quantify such as the pain and distress suffered by individuals as a result of their disability.

6. Improving the quality of care and potential savings

Ninety percent of patients with back pain recover or improve in one to three months

---

[*]Source note: Department of Social Security Figures (1993) Obtained from a 1% sample of claims for sickness and/or invalidity benefit which excluded days of incapacity where Statutory Sick Pay was claimed from the employer and most short spells of incapacity under 4 days in duration.

regardless of any treatment[18,19], although recurrences are common[4]. It is the chronic or repetitive problems that may be associated with disability and are likely to be responsible for the high cost to society. Interventions that cost-effectively reduce this disability would be advantageous. Therefore, simple forms of treatment which might speed up recovery and enable individuals to reduce the impact of recurrences appear to be the most efficient way of dealing with this sizable problem.

6.1. Self care and advice on activity

Since it is very difficult for a clinician to provide a specific diagnosis, apparently contradictory terms are used in different consultations, and labels which may be alarming are sometimes communicated to the patient. These may encourage a fear and avoidance of movement leading to further disability[20,21]. A simple non-threatening label such as back sprain has been advocated instead of terms such as arthritis, degeneration or rupture[7]. Cognitive aspects such as the meaning of the pain may have important implications for recovery, and research in this area would be worthwhile.

It has been shown that for chronic back pain patients, behavioural as well as cognitive factors are important and this is discussed further under the section heading of management of chronic pain. In a randomised controlled trial of acute back pain, Fordyce *et al.* compared traditional advice to "let pain be your guide" with a specified programme of restoration encouraging increasing activity over time[22]. No differences were found between the groups at 6 weeks follow-up on a composite variable called 'sick', but at 9-12 months follow-up the patients who had been given time-contingent advice did significantly better than those who were given traditional advice. Fordyce *et al.* reported that these findings provided evidence for the poor relationship between pain and non-healing, and also pain and physical disability which is consistent with other research reports[21].

Practice styles of primary care physicians in the US were studied in a recent quasi-experimental observational study of back pain[4]. Von Korff *et al.* found that back pain patients treated by physicians who tended to give advice on self-care measures reported significantly less limitation on activities due to pain at one month follow up than those treated by physicians who tended to prescribe medication. Although these differences were not maintained at 1-year and 2-year follow up, they also reported greater satisfaction with back care education. This study demonstrated that it is more cost-effective to encourage self-care and a resumption of activity, than to prescribe medication and bedrest.

Deyo *et al.* randomised patients with acute back pain, but no neurological deficit, to spend either 2 or 7 days in bed[23], and found that those who stayed in bed for the shorter time missed 45% fewer days of work. These authors concluded that bedrest, especially if prolonged, may be an important contributory factor in chronicity.

Linton *et al.* in another primary care study, randomised two different groups of patients with musculoskeletal disorders to traditional management versus early resumption of activities[24]. For patients who had not been on the sick list in the previous two years, early intervention was significantly more effective in reducing long term sickness compared with traditional treatment.

An alternative method of encouraging self-care may be through the use of carefully prepared education booklets. Although these abound, since most do not meet the criteria needed to ensure readability for the majority of the population[25] they may often be of limited value. There is evidence that the provision of an educational booklet can be effective in reducing General Practitioner consultations, hospital out-patient referrals and even hospital admissions and surgery[26]. There is a need to develop this type of well presented information and to find out whether it is also possible to reduce pain reports, disability and sickness absence with such a simple tool.

Some patients may benefit from being referred to a suitably qualified physiotherapist, osteopath or chiropractor. Hackett *et al.* have reported that if early physiotherapy was provided in primary care patients rated their management as above average and fewer hospital referrals resulted[27].

6.2. Spinal manipulation

There is evidence that spinal manipulation can speed up recovery in the acute stage of 2-4 weeks' onset[28,29]. Two other studies provide some evidence of the usefulness of spinal manipulation in the management of chronic back pain patients[30,31].

6.3. Exercise, and patient education

A number of randomised controlled trials have studied the effectiveness of exercise programmes for patients with back pain. Koes[32], in a blinded review of 100 papers on exercise programmes for back patients, concluded that only four studies met rigorous standards of design and were not methodologically flawed. These studies did not provide evidence of the usefulness of any particular type of exercise regimen for back pain patients, a conclusion that was also reached in other reviews of the literature[33,34]. This type of research has many problems, one of which is that the term back pain encompasses many different aetiologies, which may respond to different types of exercise, at different stages, in different individuals. It can therefore be argued that each individual needs to be assessed and exercises appropriate to that person need to be taught. This approach is not readily amenable to evaluation using a randomised controlled trial, which may account in part for the lack of evidence of the effectiveness of any one exercise regimen.

McKenzie's approach to treating back pain is currently enjoying great popularity and includes the use of passive stretching exercises and has the advantage of encouraging patients to take responsibility for their problem[35]. It has the major advantage of encouraging self-care and a sense of control. There is some evidence for its usefulness[36,37], but more research is needed to clarify its effects.

Exercise programmes that appear to be effective in improving function in chronic back pain tend to consist of quite vigorous exercises[38,39]. It can be hypothesised that patients who are given gentle exercises and told to do them avoiding any pain, may become conditioned to believe that any pain associated with movement or activity is detrimental to recovery. This could explain the negative results on pain and disability measures at 3 months in a recent large scale placebo-controlled study of a physiotherapy exercise programme for acute back pain patients[40].

Back care education programmes on their own do not necessarily appear to be effective and the results of a number of studies of back schools have been equivocal.[41] Programmes that offer a group exercise programme and encourage self care do appear to be effective[39]. Further research into the method of delivery of both exercises and education for back pain patients is needed, to find out which is the most effective.[42, 43]

There may be a role for fitness classes in primary care which aims to encourage the early resumption of physical activities, and reduce the chances of back pain patients developing chronic disabling conditions. Such a programme, based on the successful outcome of a fitness class for chronic back patients carried out in Oxford[39] is currently being set up in York and evaluated in a randomised controlled trial comparing it with standard current practice.

6.4. Referral to a radiology department

A sizable proportion of the NHS budget is taken up by radiological lumbar spine examinations, including both plain X-rays and sophisticated and expensive techniques such as Computerised Tomography (CT) and Magnetic Resonance Imaging (MRI). According to a recent study carried out in a community hospital, half of the plain lumbar spine radiographs would not have been carried out if guidelines drawn up by the Royal College of Radiologists had been followed[44-46]. The guidelines recommend that a lumbar spine radiograph is only indicated in a number of limited cases - "that is when pain is worsening or not resolving, when there is a history of trauma, or when abnormal neurological signs are evident on clinical examination"[44]. Halpin *et al.* estimated that amongst the 700,000 people who have lumbar spine radiographs each year, there is a statistical probability of up to 19 deaths occurring as a result of the radiation exposure[45].

It seems, therefore that referrals for X-rays could be reduced, benefiting patients, and at the same time providing considerable cost savings.

6.5. Hospital referrals

Referrals to out-patient clinics are not necessarily appropriate and there are large variations in referral rates[13]. In a longitudinal study of 182 GP referrals of back pain patients to outpatient clinics, Coulter *et al.*[13] found that communication between the GPs and the hospital consultants was poor. Although in only 29% of these cases, the GPs' reason for the referral was specialist treatment, in 75% of cases the outpatient referral did result in treatment. In this study referrals to radiology and physiotherapy departments were sometimes found to be duplicated following an outpatient visit.

6.6. Hospital admissions

Patients with back pain are now less frequently admitted to hospital for bedrest. However, they may still be admitted if a prolapsed intervertebral disc (PID) is suspected[47], for pain-relieving treatment such as epidural steroidal injections, or for traction. Evidence for the effectiveness of such treatments is lacking[47-50].

In-patient beds are also used for diagnostic procedures such as myelograms, which are invasive and commonly associated with side-effects. CT scans would be preferable in most cases[47]. Where an alternative can be found it is desirable to avoid hospitalisation for back pain[51].

Surgery, may have some advantages for patients with definite disc herniations and nerve root involvement[2,53], but good outcomes even in this group of patients can also result from conservative management[52]. Weber[53], in a randomised controlled trial of surgery and conservative treatment, found that 80% of patients treated conservatively showed improvement and had satisfactory outcomes at one year follow-up. At one year and four year follow-up, patients who had surgery were significantly better than those who had conservative treatment but these differences were no longer significant at ten years.

Minimally invasive surgery, such as microdiscectomies, may be the best option if surgery is indicated, such as in the case of clear cut PID. Minimally invasive surgery could potentially reduce the use of hospital beds, since patients need only stay for 24 to 48 hours[54], and speed up the rate of recovery since the operation is less traumatic. But changes in the organisation of the services would be required[55], along with specialist equipment and specialised training. Minimally invasive surgery is an example of health technology that is rapidly developing but is largely unevaluated[56]. This type of surgery is still invasive and potentially dangerous, and its use therefore needs to be closely monitored[55].

7. Managing chronic back pain

Active graded exercises, taking into account cognitive and behavioural processes such as a fear of movement which might bring on the pain, and encouraging a resumption of normal activities[20,21,39,57,58] are probably a key element in both secondary prevention and secondary care. Successful rehabilitation programmes are usually goal-oriented, use 'exercise quotas', according to the individual's baseline capacity and encourage family involvement. There is some evidence that patients who attribute their recovery to their own efforts are less likely to relapse[59].

8. Managing back pain in the workplace

Since back pain is very common amongst people who are in their most productive working years, prolonged sick leave resulting in loss of productivity is of special concern. A few studies provide some evidence that workplace interventions can be effective in reducing absenteeism due to back problems and apparently can be cost effective e.g.[60-63] They usually include ergonomic interventions, but some are based on exercise. They tend to be set up by North American or Scandinavian companies who may be more motivated to reduce medical claims, due to the differences in the benefit system compared with the UK. However, most work in this area of health promotion suffers from a number of design problems and methodological flaws. Control groups are either not included, or are unsatisfactory since contamination between the groups is likely if the workers are on the same site, and if they are not the different settings may render the groups incomparable. Also the subjects tend to be self-selected, with small numbers agreeing to participate in the programme leading to an insufficient sample size. Partly for these reasons, and also because details of the intervention and assessment procedures used are lacking, as is baseline information to allow comparison of the groups, it is difficult to analyse findings. High cost-benefits are reported in these studies but need be regarded with some scepticism. In addition, the avoidance of production losses included in the benefits lead to an exaggerated benefit figure. Although it is impossible to ascertain precisely which components are beneficial, the key to a successful programme appears to be organisational involvement[64,42,43].

The work environment has also been shown to be more important than many other physical and psychological variables in predicting individuals who are likely to report back pain[65]. There is some evidence of the important role which the supervisor in the work-place can play in helping the worker return to work. Above all the worker, who may be expected to carry out very tedious and possibly strenuous work in spite of his pain, needs to feel appreciated[65]. In any case there is evidence for the need to take into consideration psycho-social factors rather than just physical findings when assessing an individual with back pain.

9. Conclusions

One major limitation on progress at present is the difficulty of classifying different types of back pain problems. Research in this area is needed to find out which type of back pain respond to a particular approach. This is especially pertinent for exercise therapy and spinal manipulation.

However sufficient evidence has now emerged to suggest that simple management and self-care including appropriate education on back care, is the best way forward for general practice management of most acute back pain patients. Patients with neurological signs may need a slightly less aggressive approach and a physical examination to exclude these and more serious pathology is therefore necessary. This could reduce much financial expense as well as anguish due to unnecessary investigations, and inappropriate treatment.

Cost-effectiveness studies of back pain are lacking, but before they can be conducted, further research is needed to investigate which methods of treatment are most effective in both speeding up recovery and preventing recurrences.

10. Acknowledgements

Thanks are due to Trevor Sheldon for his help in analysing the data, and Dr Brenda Leese for reading the manuscript.

11. References

1.   A. White and S. Gordon, *Spine* **7** (1982) 141.
2.   R. Deyo, *Neurosurgery Clinics of North America* **2(4)** (1991) 851.
3.   V. Mooney, *J. Royal Society of Medicine* **86** (1993) 273.
4.   M. Von Korff, W. Barlow, D. Cherkin and R. Deyo, *Annals of Internal Medicine* **121** (1994) 187.

5.   H. Flor, N. Birbaumer and D. Turk, *Adv. Behav. Res. Ther.* **12** (1990) 47.
6.   G. Waddell and J. Richardson, *J. Psychosomatic Research* **36(1)** (1992) 77.
7.   G. Waddell, *Baillieres Clinical Rheumatology* **6(3)** (1992) 523.
8.   A. Frank, Education & Debate. Low Back Pain. *British Medical Journal* **306** (1993) 901.
9.   M. Roland, J. Bartholomew, M. Courtenay, R. Morris and D. Morrell, *British Medical Journal* **292** (1986) 874.
10. J. Klaber Moffett and G. Richardson, *Back Pain and its Cost to Society*. Forthcoming Discussion Paper, Centre for Health Economics, University of York 1994.
11. A. Papageorgiou, P. Croft, L. Jordan and M. Jayson, Patient consulting rates for low back pain in primary care. Society for Back Pain Research Meeting, Stoke-on-Trent, 1994.
12. J. Fry, *General Practice - The Facts* (Oxford Medical Press, Oxford, 1993)
13. A. Coulter, J. Bradlow and C. Martin-Bates, *British Journal of General Practice* **41** (1991) 450.
14. Government Statistical Service. *Hospital Episode Statistics*. Department of Health, London, 1993.
15. Proprietary Association of Great Britain. *Market Estimates 1993*. London, 1993.
16. J. Balcombe, N. Strange and G. Tate, *Wish you were here* (Industrial Society, London, 1993).
17. Confederation of British Industry. *Too Much Time Out?* (CBI,London, 1993)
18. Quebec Task Force on Spinal Disorders, W. Spitzer, F. LeBlance, M. Dupois, *et al.* Scientific approach to the assessment and management of activity-related spinal disorders: a monograph for clinicians. Quebec Task Force on Spinal Disorders. *Spine (Suppl 7)* 1987;12.
19. A.S. Dixon, *British Medical Journal* **2** (1973) 82.
20. J. Lethem, P. Slade and J. Troup, *et al.*, *Behavior Research & Therapy* **21(4)** (1983) 401.
21. G. Waddell, D. Somerville and I. Henderson, *et al.*, *Pain* **52** (1993) 157.
22. W. Fordyce, J. Brockway, J. Bergman and D. Spengler, *J. Behavioural Medicine* **9** (1986) 127.
23. R. Deyo, A. Diehl and M. Rosenthal, *The New England Journal of Medicine* **315(17)** (1986) 1064.
24. S. Linton, A.-L. Hellsing and D. Andersson, *Pain* **54** (1993) 353.
25. C. Gunn, *Primary Care Management* **3** (1993) 11.
26. M. Roland and M. Dixon, in *Back Pain - New Approaches to Education & Rehabilitation*, ed. M. Roland and J. Jenner, (Manchester University Press, 1989).
27. G. Hackett, P. Bundred, J. Hutton, J. O'Brien and I. Stanley, *British Journal of General Practice* **43** (1993) 61.
28. B. Koes, W. Assendelft and G. van der Heijden, *British Medical Journal* **303** (1991) 1298.

29. P. Shekelle, A. Adams and M. Chassin, *et al.*, *The Appropriateness of Spinal Manipulation for Low-Back Pain. Project Overview and Literature review*. Consortium for Chiropractic Research and the Foundation for Chiropractic Education and Research, 1991.

30. B. Koes, L. Bouter, M.H. Van, A. Essers, *et al.*, *British Medical Journal* **304** (1992) 601.

31. T. Meade, S. Dyer, W. Browne, J. Townsend, *et al.*, *British Medical Journal* **300** (1990) 1431.

32. B. Koes, I. Bouter, H. Beckerman, *et al.*, *British Medical Journal* **302** (1991) 1572.

33. J. Klaber Moffett, in *Back Pain - New Approaches to Rehabilitation and Education*, ed. M. Roland and J. Morris, (Manchester University Press, 1989).

34. R. Swezey and A. Petrocelli, in *The Lumbar Spine and Back Pain*. 4th edn., ed. M.I.V. Jayson (Churchill Livingstone, Edinburgh, 1992).

35. R. McKenzie, *The Lumbar Spine*. (Spinal Publications Ltd, New Zealand, 1981).

36. A. Roberts, *Conservative management of back pain. A Study of McKenzie therapy and slow release ketoprofen*. MD thesis, University of Nottingham, 1991

37. R. Stankovic and O. Johnell, *Spine* **15(2)** (1990) 120.

38. C. Manniche, E. Lundberg, I. Christensen, L. Bentzen, *et al.*, *Pain* **47** (1991) 53.

39. H. Frost, J. Klaber Moffett, J. Moser and J. Fairbank, Evaluation of a fitness programme for patients with chronic low back pain. *Submitted to British Medical Journal* (1994)

40. A. Faas, A. Chavannes, J.T.M. van Eijk and J. Gubbels, *Spine* **18** (1993) 1388.

41. B. Koes, M. van Tulder, D. van der Windt and L. Bouter, *Journal of Clinical Epidemiology* **47** (1994) 851.

42. M. Nordin, in *The Lumbar Spine & Back Pain*, 4th edn., ed. M.I.V. Jayson, (Churchill Livingstone, Edinburgh, 1992).

43. R. Deyo, D. Cherkin, D. Conrad and E. Volinn, *Annual Review Public Health* **12** (1991) 141.

44. Royal College of Radiologists. *Making the best use of a Department of Radiology: Guidelines for doctors*. RCR, London, 1989.

45. S. Halpin, L. Yeoman and D. Dundas, *British Medical Journal* **303** (1991) 813.

46. R. Chisholm, *British Medical Journal* **303** (1991) 797.

47. M. Deane, A. Moore, A. Long and S. Harrison, *A study to identify current treatment and audit activity in relation to the prolapsed lumbar intervertebral disc*. Nuffield Institute for Health, Leeds, 1993.

48. J. Cuckler, A. Nada and L. Rymaskewski, *J Bone Joint Surg.* **67-A** (1985) 63.

49. B. Pal, P. Mangion, M. Hossain and B. Diffey, *British Journal of Rheumatology* **25** (1986) 181.
50. R. Deyo, J. Loeser and S. Bigos, *Annals of Internal Medicine* **112** (1990) 598.
51. D. Cherkin and R. Deyo, *Spine* **18** (1993) 1728.
52. J. Saal and J. Saal, *Spine* **14** (1989) 431.
53. H. Weber, *Spine* **8** (1983) 131.
54. R. Deyo, D. Cherkin, J. Loeser, *et al.*, *J. Bone Joint Surg.* **74**-**A** (1992) 536.
55. H. Banta, *British Medical Journal* **307** (1993) 1546.
56. R. Smith, *British Medical Journal* **307** (1993) 1403.
57. I. Lindstrom, C. Ohlund, C. Eek, L. Wallin, L. Petersson, W. Fordyce *et al.*, *Physical Therapy* **72(4)** (1992) 279.
58. A.C. Williams, M.K. Nicholas, P.H. Richardson, *et al.*, *British Journal of General Practice* **43** (1993) 513.
59. J. Dolce, M. Crocker, Moletierre and D. Doleys, *Pain* **24** (1986) 365.
60. R. Todd Brown, B. Page and P. McMahan, *Human Factors Society Bulletin* **34** (1991) 1.
61. S. Leiyu, *Public Health* **108** (1993) 204.
62. K. Brown, A. Sirles, J. Hilyer and M. Thomas, *Spine* **17** (1992) 1224.
63. B. Gundewall, M. Liljeqvist and T. Hansson, *Spine* **18** (1993) 587.
64. D. Wood, *Spine* **12(2)** (1987) 77.
65. S. Bigos, M. Battié, D. Spengler, *et al.*, *Spine* **16(1)** (1991) 1.

Index

acceleration 12, 15, 17, 32
adolescent 164, 179
aetiology 51, 97
ageing 4, 46, 52, 55, 105
aggrecan 51-56, 63, 76
anatomy 1, 3, 8, 9, 73, 74, 85, 94, 134
angiogenesis 94
angiography 208, 220
ankylosing spondylitis 132
annulus fibrosus 5, 9, 27, 53-55, 57, 58, 64, 74, 78, 80, 81, 85, 88, 89, 92, 93, 132,
    185
antibiotic 175
antibodies 73, 79-81, 142
aorta 210, 212, 214, 222
arachnoiditis 133
arch 1-11, 27
arthrodesis 184, 185

bending 1-4, 7-12, 15-23, 28, 35, 44, 45, 73,
bending moment 3, 4, 7, 8, 11, 12, 16, 18-22
biglycan 57-59
biopsy 141, 208, 211, 212, 217, 219, 221
blood
    flow 86, 89, 90, 93, 94, 115-118, 127-129, 134, 142, 220
    supply 68, 79, 115, 210, 216, 220
    vessels 76, 80, 87-91, 93, 94, 133, 140, 142
body weight 12, 15, 27, 66, 67, 116
bone graft 214
buckling 109

calcification 65, 80-82, 178, 179
calcitonin gene related peptide 80, 85, 86
cauda equina 97, 103, 120, 122, 124-129, 131, 134, 163, 165, 175, 179-181
cells 54, 57-60, 63, 65-69, 71, 74-80, 82, 91-94, 117, 133, 135, 136, 141-143
chemonucleolysis 163-168, 173, 175-183
chondrocyte 136
chondroitin sulphate 52, 54-58, 74
chymopapain 163, 166, 169, 172, 177-180
clavicle 99
collagen 5, 6, 9, 52, 57-59, 64, 65, 74-78, 81, 82, 91, 94, 107, 109, 142, 164
compensation 144, 146, 148-152, 178, 196, 197
complications 163, 166, 169, 175, 180, 188, 202, 208, 216, 220, 223

computer tomography 97, 102, 109, 123, 132, 145, 152, 163, 168, 177, 191, 193,
    208-210, 229
conservative treatment 163, 230
cost 155, 164, 225-227, 229
creep 20, 22, 48
cricket 23
curvature 1, 2, 4, 5, 8, 10, 12, 18
cytokines 65, 68, 77, 92, 142

damping 32-35
decompression 27, 179, 205, 218, 221
decorin 57-59
deformity 30, 38, 39, 92, 216, 220
depression 117, 152, 157, 158, 160, 200
diabetes 105
diffusion 53, 69, 79, 81, 115, 133
discography 107-109, 169, 178, 189, 191-193, 197, 198, 200, 204
dura 97, 130, 172, 173, 208, 212-214, 216, 220, 221
dynamics 12, 109, 126

education 154, 161, 162, 224, 227-229, 231-233
efficiency 10
emg 17, 18, 129
endplate 47-49, 67, 73, 75-77, 79-83, 89, 92, 94, 140, 186, 189
enzyme 79, 163, 164, 166
equilibrium 3-5, 7, 10, 12, 29-31
erector spinae 1, 6, 12, 16, 18, 22, 111, 214
exercise 63-65, 69, 119, 122, 129, 132, 145, 160, 228, 230, 231
extension catch 28, 33, 35, 145
extracellular matrix 51, 53, 54, 58, 60, 63

facet joint 48, 87, 105, 109, 111, 116, 145, 148, 184-189, 192, 193, 198
facetectomy 187, 192, 205
fatigue 12, 15, 20, 22, 23, 25, 39, 40, 157, 201, 219
fear 154, 158-160, 227, 230
fibromodulin 57, 59
fissure 107, 109, 111-113
fitness 65, 156, 160, 229, 233
fixation 38, 91, 185, 207, 208, 216, 219
flexibility 1, 2, 8, 12, 30, 42, 63, 81
foetus 57, 103
force 2-5, 7, 8, 10-12, 15-18, 22, 23, 29, 30, 32-36, 65, 111, 112, 155, 161, 204, 232
functional nucleus 46-48
funicular polygon 2

fusion 39, 64, 87, 88, 149-151, 165, 185, 186, 191, 193, 196, 197, 204, 205, 207, 219, 221
general practice 159, 224, 225, 231, 232, 234
glucose 64, 65, 69, 86
glycogen 64
glycosaminoglycan 51, 52, 57-59, 76, 82
Graf implant 184, 204, 205
gymnastics 23

Harrington rod 39
Hartshill horseshoe 39
Hartshill rectangle 39-41, 216
health resources 224
hyaluronan 52-57
hydraulic amplifier 9
hydrostatic pressure 43, 45, 67, 68, 107, 112
hypermobility 185, 188, 204, 205

iliocostalis lumborum 6-8
implant 39-41, 184, 186, 192, 204, 205
in situ hybridisation 141, 142
inappropriate signs 120, 146, 149
inertia 32, 33, 35
infection 27, 165, 175, 180, 181, 192, 198, 204, 205
inflammation 92-94, 132, 135, 143
innervation 5, 8, 12, 80, 82, 85, 87-89, 91, 92, 186, 191
instability 26-28, 30, 33, 35, 36, 149, 187, 189, 192, 193, 196
intervertebral disc 19, 35, 42, 43, 45, 47, 48, 52, 54, 57-60, 63, 64, 67, 73, 74, 76-80, 82, 85, 88, 89, 91, 93, 94, 105, 109, 115, 117, 118, 132, 136, 144, 156, 166, 177, 181, 229, 233
    coccygeal 66
    prolapsed 22, 46, 48, 49, 132, 133, 143, 144, 146, 163-165, 193, 197
    sequestrated 165
intra-abdominal pressure 2, 3, 6, 10-12, 16
intradiscal pressure 48, 69, 89, 179
ischaemia 92, 139, 141-143
Isotrak 19

keratan sulphate 52, 55-57, 59, 77

lactic acid 64, 65, 68, 143
leg length 99
lever 2, 3, 7, 8, 10, 16, 22, 111
lifting 1-3, 9, 10, 12, 15-17, 19, 20, 22, 25, 156, 158

ligament 35, 47, 67, 75, 111, 112,
    anterior longitudinal 5, 88
    interspinous 5
    Graf (see Graf implant)
    healing 94
    posterior longitudinal 5, 22, 88, 105, 213
    supraspious 6, 88
    spondylolysis 90
ligamentum flavum 6, 88, 91, 92, 97, 120, 173, 187
link protein 52, 56
local authority 224, 226
locking 188
longissimus thoracis 6-8
lordosis 4, 10-12, 188, 202
lumbar instability syndrome 187, 189, 192, 193, 196
lumican 57, 59
Luque 38, 40, 195

macrophage 94
magnetic resonance imaging 65, 97, 99, 117, 118, 121, 132, 152, 163, 164, 190, 192,
    193, 197, 198, 200, 208, 209, 210, 212, 219, 221, 229
McKenzie 228, 233
microsphere 115, 116, 118, 119
motion segment 19, 22, 23, 109, 113, 144, 149, 184, 186-188, 191, 192, 199, 200,
    204, 205
MRI (see magnetic resonance imaging)
mRNA 55, 57, 141, 142
multifidus 8
myelography 133, 135, 163, 169, 208

nerve conduction 130, 134
nerve root 98, 105, 109, 129, 132-136, 138, 142, 143, 145, 172, 187, 210, 216, 222,
    229
neurogenic claudication 97, 119-123, 128-130, 144, 145
neuropathology 122
neuropeptide 80, 82, 85-92, 94, 195
neuropeptide Y 85-92, 94
newborn 53-55
nucleus pulposus 42, 52, 53, 55, 57, 59, 64, 67, 74, 77, 78, 80, 89, 91, 92, 106, 133,
    166, 169, 172, 173
nutrition 65, 79, 81, 89, 115, 117

obesity 156
osteoarthritis 71
osteophyte 135, 137, 138, 179

osteoporosis 196
osteotomy 209, 212, 221
oxygen 17, 64, 68, 69, 115, 118, 133

pain drawing 197
papain 163
pedicle screw 39, 186, 199, 205, 214
pedicles 97, 100, 103, 104, 116, 213, 217, 219, 221
periosteum 85, 90, 136
Perthes disease 115
PET (see positron emission tomography)
pH 68
physiotherapy 163, 167, 206, 225, 228, 229
positron emission tomography 115, 118, 119, 129
posture 2, 4, 5, 7, 8, 10, 12, 27, 28, 30, 33, 46, 47, 120, 132, 189
pregnancy 164
prescriptions 225
prostaglandin 92, 94
proteoglycan 5, 49, 51-59, 63-68, 74-79, 82, 94, 164
protrusion 97, 98, 104, 105, 122, 137, 138, 173, 175, 178, 179, 181
pseudarthrosis 151, 221
psoas major 9

radiculography 122 -126, 132
radiology 153, 163, 223, 225, 229, 233
reconstruction 208, 212, 214, 219
reflex arc 129, 131
revision 204
root entrapment 97, 104, 120, 168

sciatica 105, 133, 144, 156, 166-168, 178, 182, 193, 194
scoliosis 4, 39, 41, 65, 73, 74, 76, 77, 79-83, 88, 92, 122, 123, 125, 127, 186, 187
self care 227, 228
shear 9, 11, 12, 15, 17, 18, 23, 27, 28, 43, 45, 47, 109
sickle-cell anaemia 117, 119
skull 99, 103
smoking 134, 148, 156
spina bifida 102, 104
spinal probing 206
spondylolisthesis 12, 27, 28, 35, 109, 122, 123, 125, 132, 146, 149, 178, 184-186, 196
spondylolysis 23, 90, 91, 94, 102-104, 149
stabilisation 184, 186, 191-193, 196, 197, 199, 204-206, 208, 214-216, 218, 219, 221
stability 2-4, 6, 9-12, 14, 26, 29, 30, 32, 36, 44, 55, 56, 186-188, 204
stanozolol 134
stenosis 102, 104, 120-125, 127-132, 164, 178, 187

straight leg raising 8, 10, 156, 157, 163, 168, 169, 178
strain gauge 39, 40, 42, 43
stress profile 43, 45-47, 49, 191
substance P 80, 85-94
sulphate 52, 54-59, 64, 69, 74, 77, 79

thoracolumbar fascia 2, 3, 6, 7, 9, 11, 12
torsion 15, 19, 20
training 166, 224, 230
trauma 27, 133, 142, 145, 156, 183, 223, 225, 229
tumour 27, 122, 208, 210-214, 216-222
twist test 193

ultrasound 97, 178

vacuum effect 107
vasoactive intestinal peptide 80, 85, 86
velocity 17, 18, 32
venous congestion 122, 126-128, 134
vertebral body 22, 79, 81, 85, 90, 99, 109, 112, 113, 115, 117-119, 174, 187, 20⁵
    209, 213, 214, 216-218
vertebral canal 97, 99, 101, 103, 104, 120, 129
vibration 20, 65, 67, 115
viscoelastic 5, 35
von Willebrand factor 141

water 51, 63, 64, 74, 75, 78, 82, 115, 118, 168, 169
workplace 15, 230